WOMEN OF ROCHESTER PEDIATRICS

WOMEN OF ROCHESTER PEDIATRICS

IN THEIR OWN WORDS

Nancy Wharton Bolger

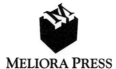

MELIORA PRESS

An imprint of the University of Rochester Press

First published 2019

University of Rochester Press
668 Mt. Hope Avenue, Rochester, NY 14620, USA
www.urpress.com
and Boydell & Brewer Limited
PO Box 9, Woodbridge, Suffolk IP12 3DF, UK
www.boydellandbrewer.com

ISBN-13: 978-1-58046-948-7

Library of Congress Cataloging-in-Publication Data

Names: Bolger, Nancy W., author.
Title: Women of Rochester pediatrics : in their own words / Nancy Wharton Bolger.
Description: Rochester, NY : Meliora Press, an imprint of the University of Rochester Press, 2019.
Identifiers: LCCN 2019013903 | ISBN 9781580469487 (pbk. : alk. paper)
Subjects: | MESH: University of Rochester. School of Medicine and Dentistry. | Pediatricians | Physicians, Women | Schools, Medical | New York | Biography
Classification: LCC RJ43.A1 | NLM WZ 112.5.P3 | DDC 618.9200092/274789—dc23 LC record available at https://lccn.loc.gov/2019013903

This publication is printed on acid-free paper.
Printed in the United States of America.

This volume is dedicated to
Roger and Carolyn Friedlander,
friends of all children.

CONTENTS

PREFACE

"Optimism is the faith that leads to achievement. Nothing can be done without hope and confidence."

—Helen Keller (1880–1968)

In *Women of Rochester Pediatrics: In Their Own Words*, twenty-nine remarkable women, most of whom are professors of pediatrics at the University of Rochester School of Medicine and Dentistry, relate the history of their lives in their own words. All have built impressive careers while weaving social lives rich with the pleasures of family, friends, and community. They share personal advice as women on how to negotiate a career in the complex world of medicine. This advice is relevant to our male colleagues as well as to colleagues in other professions.

As each recounts her story, through interviews with the author, one hears similar themes of "optimism, hope, and confidence" despite many professional and personal challenges. At such times, these women remained optimistic, and hoped to achieve their dreams of being a doctor even though when most trained, there was a paucity of women in the profession that further increased their challenge. They persisted in pursuit of their careers despite adversity. They were confident in their abilities to meet their professional pursuits and had faith that they would achieve their dreams even if it took more time than originally planned. Most were high-achieving from an early age and were willing to spend many years in rigorous and prolonged higher education. All express love of service to children and gratitude for those who supported them through life's journey: families, mentors, colleagues, and trainees. Indeed despite the ups and downs of their professional pursuits, combining careers and family, they persisted. Contemporary youth must not be discouraged or be persuaded by others not to pursue their dreams. In life, there are many joys and challenges, and achieving one's dreams can be accomplished with optimism, hope, and confidence.

In 1968, when I arrived at the University of Rochester, the Department of Pediatrics was forty years old—and listed no female professors of pediatrics on its faculty. Not until the mid- to late 1980s were three nationally recognized women promoted to full professor. For many years, we constituted a single-digit percentage of freshman medical school classes.

Today, as issues relating to gender equity are debated nationally, academic medicine is experiencing cultural shifts similar to those occurring in the larger world. We celebrate the gender equality that has been achieved—gradually—in admissions to US medical schools. In 2017, more women than men were admitted to the nation's medical schools (50.7 percent).[1] The same equity, however, has not permeated the highest levels of leadership in academic medical centers, where only 16 percent of medical school deans are now women.[2] However, at the University of Rochester, two women in succession have recently chaired our Department spanning the past quarter of a century. Currently 57 percent of our department's Executive Cabinet are women, a clear sign of changing times.

As we celebrate the accomplishments of these twenty-nine remarkable women, we also honor all the women physicians across the country, those in both full-time academic medicine and those in practice, who have bravely faced and overcome multiple career challenges, often alone. After many years, these dedicated women continue to be energized by their primary mission: serving and advocating for the best interests of children and families.

This book is dedicated to Roger and Carolyn Friedlander. Mr. Friedlander, a graduate of the University of Rochester, was chair of the Board of Golisano Children's Hospital and is a member of the University of Rochester's Board of Trustees. He has been devoted to our university, the Department of Pediatrics, and its children's hospital for nearly three decades. Mrs. Friedlander was a member of the inaugural class of nurse practitioners at the University of Rochester School of Nursing and practiced pediatrics for twenty-five years at Rochester's Elmwood Pediatrics Group. In addition, she is an active volunteer at the university's Memorial Art Gallery. The Friedlander family's support over many years has allowed the expansion of many programs in pediatrics; they and their family are all special "friends of children."

As pediatricians, we look to future generations of young people continuing the great work of their predecessors in caring for and improving the lives of children and adolescents. The voices of the women who speak in the following pages make us both proud of them and optimistic for the future. We know many younger women who are already hard at work building strong academic careers and clinical practices, enjoying life, and always advocating for the best interests of children and their families at the same time that they are facing the fast-changing world in which we live. Meliora!

Elizabeth R. McAnarney, MD

Notes

Epigraph: Helen Keller, *Optimism: An Essay* (1903).

1. *AAMC News*, "More Women Than Men Enrolled in U.S. Medical Schools in 2017," December 18, 2017.

2. Travis, Elizabeth, *AAMC News*, "Academic Medicine Needs More Women Leaders," January 16, 2018.

ACKNOWLEDGEMENTS

I would like to thank each of the women faculty who participated in this project. Without them, there would be no book—and one less addition to our department's archival history. Author Nancy Wharton Bolger, who also wrote the companion history, *Rochester Pediatrics*, spent many hours talking with the participants, recording the interviews, crafting each chapter, editing and reediting. Carole Berger, with whom I have worked for forty-four years, has been the bridge between Nancy and me as she coordinated many moving parts with her usual grace. Martha Preston, our departmental administrative colleague, skillfully oversaw the administrative details associated with the project. We also acknowledge Sonia Kane and Susan Smith of the University of Rochester Press for their contributions to this volume.

I would be remiss if I didn't acknowledge several male colleagues who have a special ability to mentor both women and men. They represent many other men who are advocating for equity for women in medical school. The late Dr. Robert A. Hoekelman was the chair of pediatrics who nominated the first three women for professorships in the mid-1980s; he also created several programs to support young female residents. I would like to especially acknowledge Drs. Francis Gigliotti, Christopher Hodgman, Richard Kreipe, Thomas McInerny, David Siegel, and Peter Szilagyi for their outstanding mentorship of women (and men). I would like also to acknowledge the late Dr. Augusta B. McCoord (1897–1979), an unsung heroine of our department, who served children hospitalized at the Strong Memorial Hospital by singlehandedly running the Department of Pediatrics's chemistry laboratory twenty-four hours a day for thirty-five years.

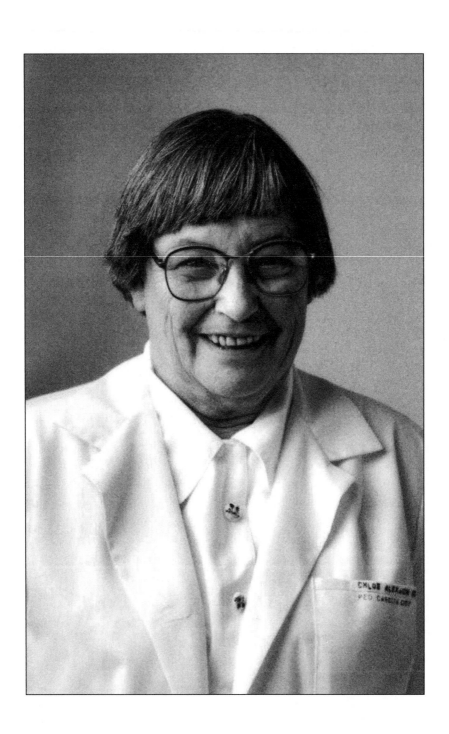

Chapter One

Chloe G. Alexson, MD (1928-2014)[1]

Cardiologist Chloe Alexson is remembered as one of the most revered teachers in the long history of the University of Rochester Medical Center (URMC). Honors were bestowed on this beloved teacher with impressive regularity: seventeen awards in near-consecutive years during the 1980s and '90s. The most treasured, her close colleagues believe, were the prizes awarded by the students in the medical classes and pediatric resident trainees to whom she had introduced the heart's complexities.

A major national award came in 1986, when the American Heart Association named Dr. Alexson "Teacher of the Year" on the subject of cardiovascular diseases. Her regard by the University she served was made clear in 1993 when she was presented with the University of Rochester Alumni Association's Gold Medal Award in recognition of her "integrity, inspiring teaching, and devotion to medical students."

Perhaps a better sense of who Chloe Alexson was can be found in an essay she wrote toward the end of her career. In it, she speaks of her hopes for young people about to begin their careers: "I hope that when they're my age, they bound out of bed in the morning eager to go to work, as I still am. Every morning I thank God that I knew what I wanted to be when I grew up—and that I was right."

Chloe was born in 1928 in the small town of Oradell, New Jersey. While none in her immediate family were engaged in the medical profession, she seems to have known from an early age that she wanted to be a doctor. After graduating from Cornell University in 1950, she pursued that goal, despite the strong resistance of most medical schools to educating women physicians. She later told her story in a letter published in the University of Rochester (UR) alumni magazine:

> Even the medical school interviewers didn't change my mind. "My God! Another female! Why don't you go home and have babies?" That, of course, was not my experience at the University of Rochester, where I still remember with pleasure all of my interviews, discussing baseball with Dr. Bradford [then chair of pediatrics], ecology (a brand new idea) with Dr. Hermann Bahn, having tea with Dean Whipple, and most of all being greeted by name and as if I mattered . . . I wouldn't and couldn't have gone to any other school.

In 1954, following her medical school graduation, Dr. Alexson became, in succession, a rotating intern, assistant resident, and associate resident at UR. In 1966, she was awarded a two-year fellowship to support the new Division of Pediatric Cardiology. As the division's first clinical fellow and later as assistant professor in the Department of Pediatrics, she worked closely with founding chief, Dr. James Manning, who had been recruited from Johns Hopkins.

Pediatric cardiology as a subspecialty was in its infancy at that time. Dramatic advances in surgical correction of congenital heart problems required the skills of a team of pediatric cardiologists. As chief, much of Dr. Manning's time during those early years was spent developing a nationally recognized program that emphasized a whole-team approach to managing treatment and care for children with heart problems.

"Chloe became the rock that sustained the local program," says Dr. Manning, "while I worked to expand patient services throughout central, western, and northern New York. Chloe had an intense interest in taking care of people. Her dedication to students, residents, and house staff was exceptional, and she was a tremendous support to me." Drs. Manning and Alexson made an impressive team, and their efforts were soon strengthened by the arrival of J. Peter Harris, MD, a graduate of Stanford University and UR's School of Medicine and Dentistry.

From the medical school's beginning in 1925, research and clinical care have been equally valued. An unattributed reminiscence in the alumni journal notes: "Those who worked alongside [Dr. Alexson] knew from the early going that she possessed tremendous clinical talent. But it was the extraordinary way that she would connect with her patients—staying after hours to watch over them and crying with them when they lost a child—that those around her continued to remember."

Dr. Harris says, "Chloe taught me that each child was a mystery unto itself that needed to be solved, and she showed me how to go about it in a caring manner. That's why many of her patients kept in touch with her long after she retired."

Dr. Alexson's outstanding talent as a teacher was soon recognized. She relished the opportunity to share both her knowledge and love for her subject. During her lectures, she scorned using slides and, later, PowerPoint; instead, she leaned into the microphone and addressed her audience directly, speaking entirely from memory. A tough, but fair, instructor, she was always clear about her expectations. "There's no question in my mind that she was one of the very best teachers I had during my pediatric residency," says Elise van der Jagt, MD, MPH, UR chief of the Division of Pediatric Hospital Medicine.

A record remains of Dr. Alexson's success in mentoring second-year pediatric residents in how to evaluate and present patients' medical records. Included among the students' post-lecture comments are these: "Knowing how to present well is a necessary skill and Dr. Alexson gave some great points in the Do's and Don'ts of formal presentations." "The best part was hearing that discharge summaries could be and should be limited to one page." And "Dr. Alexson is always encouraging [and] inspirational."

Dr. Alexson's long tenure spanned numerous changes in clinical care and many technological advances. But while she realized the benefits that came with the new tools, she continued to worry that they were replacing physicians' ability to diagnose patients using their own diagnostic skills. A hands-on physician, she would use technology to confirm what she had learned from the physical exam. "If I had my way," she told one sonographer, "you wouldn't have a job. We use Echo [echocardiography] too much."

Dr. Alexson's contributions to the medical literature were numerous. She was first author on publications related to a community rheumatic fever prophylaxis program; acute rheumatic fever; and pulmonic stenosis. Subjects of other papers for which she was co-author included trials of a vaccine in high-risk infants; risk in long-term post-surgical use of Warfarin following cardiac valve replacement in children; and Respiratory Syncytial Virus (RSV) infection in children with congenital heart disease.

Within her profession, she was a member of Alpha Omega Alpha, the Genesee Valley Heart Association, and the UR Medical Alumni Association. Within the local medical community, she served as a consultant in pediatric cardiology at Rochester General Hospital, the Genesee Hospital, and Olean General Hospital. After retiring, she continued to volunteer in the medical school's alumni office. The Dr. Chloe Alexson Scholarship Award enables an outstanding emergency service worker to attend a two-day professional training conference.

Dr. Alexson and her husband, William, a member of the medical staff at the Eastman Kodak Co., had three children. Timothy is an attorney in Mendon, New York; Peter is a retired recreational therapist in Rochester; and Andrew is a minister and online professor in Tennessee. Despite her rigorous hours at the medical center, from 6 a.m. to 6 p.m. and often through the night, Chloe was an avid reader and gardener. Every day, she quickly worked through the *New York Times* crossword puzzle, Dr. Manning recalls.

"Chloe was the consummate role model for caring," says Dr. Harris. "Although the glass-ceiling and inequitable pay rates were firmly in place, Chloe worked harder than most of the male faculty. Using only the tools then available—stethoscope, EKG, X-ray, and cardiac catheterization—she used her innate diagnostic skills to work wonders."

Dr. Chloe Alexson is a woman to be remembered and honored.

Note

1. Author's thanks to J. Peter Harris, MD, trainee and colleague of Dr. Alexson, for sharing much of the information on which this profile is based.

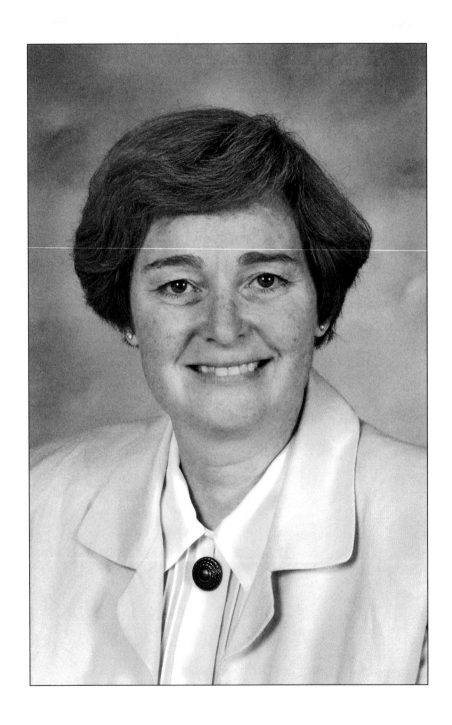

Chapter Two

BARBARA L. ASSELIN, MD

In 2009, Dr. Barbara Lawrence Asselin, long a professor of both pediatrics and hematology/oncology, changed careers. Well known for her work with national cancer trials and as a teacher, Dr. Asselin became a hospitalist at the University of Rochester's new Golisano Children's Hospital. With that, she joined what is now the fastest-growing medical subspecialty in the US, with thirty thousand members.

The career of "hospitalist" was unknown when young Barbara Lawrence received her medical degree from the UR School of Medicine and Dentistry in 1981. Over the next decades, as the ever-changing practice of medicine rolled on, tightened hospital budgets resulted in dramatic changes in patient care. Stringent limits were set on hospital admissions; only those with acute illness or serious injury in need of specialized care were admitted as inpatients. At the same time, community doctors, faced with similar fiscal constraints, realized that packed appointment schedules left them with no time to see their hospitalized patients.

As a result, hospital management recruited physicians trained in specialized clinical care to oversee the fast-paced, time-consuming management of hospitalized patients.

"Becoming a hospitalist came late in my career," Dr. Asselin says and notes jokingly that she may be "the oldest member of the youngest medical specialty." What she finds most compelling are her new patients, children with complex medical conditions that often involve multiple organ systems, too complicated for their own doctor to manage.

As Dr. Asselin's career has evolved, it has become multifaceted. In addition to the long hours she spends with patients, she is a research investigator on several national and international clinical trials. Chief among them is directing the UR component of a Dana-Farber Cancer Institute multi-site study of ways to prevent and treat leukemia. She also instructs residents, fellows, and junior faculty, as do her faculty colleagues.

Barbara grew up in a family where practicing medicine at a high level was a given. Both her parents are doctors. Her mother, Dr. Ruth Lawrence, is another "woman of Rochester Pediatrics," profiled in Chapter 20 of this book—a nationally renowned pediatrician and lactation specialist, author of the "bible" that helped transform the way new mothers fed their babies, rejecting formula-based bottle-feeding in favor of breastfeeding. Her father, Dr. Robert Lawrence, was a renowned anesthesiologist, a UR professor of anesthesiology, and founder of the American Board for Respiratory Therapy.

"I was always going to be a doctor," she says. "I came to it early because I saw it at home." As the second eldest of nine children, Barbara also learned a lot about what it means to take care of children. At St. Thomas More School in Rochester and later Our Lady of Mercy High School, she excelled in mathematics and science and discovered that she loved problem-solving.

At Boston College (BC), she found a group of men and women undergraduates who would become her lifelong "best friends." "BC was the right school for me," she says. "I loved it, and I met my husband there at the first freshman mixer!" Although only a quarter of the students in her pre-med courses were women, she was never without female friends; there were many women in her core classes, drawn to the college's undergraduate and graduate nursing programs, as well as its school of education.

Barbara graduated from Boston College in 1977 with a degree in science, *summa cum laude*. At that time, the situation for young people beginning their graduate studies was challenging. Many institutions of higher learning were seeking to diversify their student population, an outreach that came to be known as "affirmative action." ("White men," including Barbara's best friend and soon-to-be husband, Dennis Asselin, faced the toughest odds, she says.) Even students with excellent marks faced stiff competition for medical school admission.

"We were advised to apply to fifteen or twenty medical schools," Dr. Asselin recalls, "and we considered ourselves fortunate if we had two or three acceptances. Even 'legacy' didn't matter. Dennis and I were seriously dating, but there was little or no chance we would be accepted by the same school"; they weren't. Barbara chose the University of Rochester; Dennis stayed in Massachusetts at Boston University. "Every month his phone bill [to Barbara in Rochester] was about $200," she recalls, "even though we wrote to each other almost every day." Fortunately, Dennis was able to transfer to Rochester and finish his third and fourth years of medical school in Rochester, and they soon married.

"I always thought I'd be a pediatrician," says Dr. Asselin. "I had all those brothers and sisters to help care for and I also babysat. I love kids!" She says she also loved every one of her third-year medical school clinical rotations, and she appreciated the way medicine was taught at UR in those days. During the first semester, students were divided into groups of four, with one female student in each group. "We stayed together, even in lab classes, for the first two years," she recalls. "We spent the hours from 8 a.m. to 5 p.m. in the classroom, and Thursday afternoons were free. Spending all that time together, we really bonded."

During her medical student days, Barbara met Dr. Harvey Cohen, then UR's chief of pediatric hematology. Dr. Cohen, who later became chair of the Department of Pediatrics at Stanford University, had a profound effect on trainees and attracted a number of medical students into the field of pediatric hematology/oncology. Barbara was one of them.

The Drs. Asselin—Barbara and Dennis—graduated together on the same stage, receiving their medical degrees from the University of Rochester in 1981. All eleven members of the immediate Lawrence family were there to applaud and cheer on the new graduates.

In 1981, Dr. Barbara Asselin began her pediatrics internship and residency at the University of Massachusetts (UMass) Medical Center in Worcester. Although there was no "couples matching" for medical students in those days, a letter from UR Dean Douglas Angevine made it possible for Barbara and Dennis to "match" together, she in pediatrics, he in internal medicine.

The chair of pediatrics at UMass at that time was Dr. J. Barry Hanshaw, a former UR Department of Pediatrics faculty member who later became dean of the UMass medical school. "[At UMass] I shadowed a young woman who had trained under Harvey Cohen, my memorable UR professor," Dr. Asselin recalls. "She was in her first faculty position and I could see how good she was at her job, so upbeat. I thought, 'Yes! I want to be like her.'" Dr. Asselin also realized how fascinating cancer science is and how powerful the relationship doctors have with their patients can be. Dr. Asselin excelled as a pediatrics intern and resident at UMass and graduated to become Dr. Hanshaw's chief resident.

After completing her residency in 1984, Dr. Asselin returned to Rochester to begin her faculty career as instructor in pediatrics and fellow in pediatric hematology/oncology with Harvey Cohen. "After a few experiences when I dissolved in a puddle of tears, I came to realize what a wonderful specialty 'hem/onc' is," she says, using the medical slang term for hematology/oncology. Through him, she made her research connection with the Dana-Farber Cancer Institute, an important piece of mentoring with far-reaching results.

From 1996 to 2010, Dr. Asselin was principal investigator for the UR Program in the Pediatric Oncology Group, which was part of a merger in 2000 of four pediatric clinical trials' groups eventuating in the Children's Oncology Group (COG), an international consortium of more than 200 children's hospitals involved in clinical trials and the treatment of childhood cancer sponsored by the National Cancer Institute.

In 2009, Dr. Asselin realized that although she enjoyed teaching and research, something was missing. After a period of self-examination, she saw the answer. "I needed to be involved in providing direct clinical care to patients who need it. That's what I do best," she says. Since then, she has worked as an attending pediatric hospitalist at Golisano Children's Hospital at Strong while continuing to participate in and conduct clinical trials as a member of both COG and the Dana-Farber Institute Leukemia Consortium.

That she's not only succeeding in her new post but is helping others is a view supported by one of her research mentees, Dr. Keely Dwyer-Matzky, a medicine/pediatric hospitalist and director of Highland Hospital's Observation Unit. "Barbara spent many hours helping me work through the complexities of a four-year research project and she patiently reviewed multiple versions of my first manuscript. She's provided both life and career guidance, from job negotiating to work-life balance issues. I'm fortunate to have her as mentor, colleague, and friend."

Dr. Asselin is another of the Department of Pediatrics faculty women who successfully combine career and family. She and her husband, an ophthalmologist in private practice, have raised three boys. Rob, the eldest, is an engineer currently working on an expansion of LaGuardia Airport. Patrick is a pediatric neurology resident at Boston Children's Hospital carrying on the Lawrence family's medical tradition. The youngest, Michael, who had heart failure when he was eighteen months old, is now working on his master's degree in occupational therapy in Buffalo.

For young women considering a career in medicine, Dr. Asselin has the following advice:

- Research job expectations. ("They're not what they used to be.")
- Become competent in both typing and computer skills. ("You'll probably be your own secretary!")
- Learn to be flexible.
- If you're planning a family, prepare ahead for an effective daycare system. ("You have to have help!")
- Turn to friends and family for support—and be ready to reciprocate.

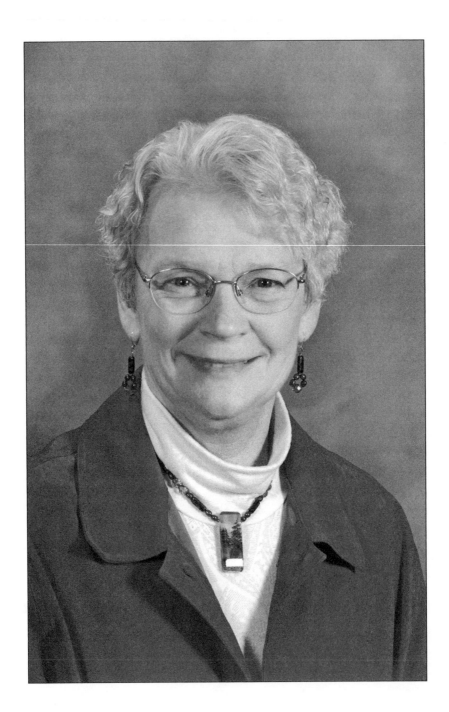

Chapter Three

CONSTANCE D. BALDWIN, PhD

Dr. Constance Baldwin is an anomaly—a professor of pediatrics who never went to medical school. Her bachelor's, master's and doctoral degrees are in English literature and language. She can tell you all about Shakespeare's use of classical rhetoric, but she never did a medical residency.

So why is Dr. Baldwin here at the University of Rochester in the Department of Pediatrics? Because, at this moment in modern history, our ability to use the English language with expertise and to a purpose is ebbing and Dr. Baldwin has spent her career fighting to reverse that trend. She is a doctor of a special kind: someone who teaches doctors, nurses, medical students, and bioscientists how to communicate with clarity, how to develop programs that meet their intended goals, and how to become educational scholars and leaders.

Dr. Baldwin's targeted faculty workshops address specific problems: how to write clearly about science, how to write grants that have the best chance of being funded, and how to develop strategies for career advancement. Whatever the topic, participants learn to identify their target message and communicate it succinctly and effectively. As clarity of language improves, confusion diminishes. Everyone gains.

The woman who anticipated a career teaching Shakespeare at an Ivy League university unexpectedly changed course years ago. Now her classroom is national as she consults at universities and health/science centers, teaching career skills required to meet the challenges of twenty-first-century healthcare.

"I have academic blood in my veins," Dr. Baldwin says. Her father, Dr. Alfred Baldwin, was a world-famous developmental psychologist and chair of his department at Cornell University in Ithaca, New York. Advanced degrees were the rule on both sides of her family.

Because young Connie Baldwin herself was intellectually gifted, she often felt out of step with her classmates. "Being different is something I've had to deal with my whole life. I was lucky to grow up in a university town," Dr. Baldwin says. Ithaca's public schools had high standards, and Connie was a prize-winning student with a gift for languages. Her future seemed clear: She would become a teacher. After all, teaching was what the Baldwin family did, often at an exalted level.

At Oregon's Reed College, Connie received excellent grounding in science, as well as in her special interest, English language and literature of the Renaissance. She graduated Phi Beta Kappa in 1968, and over the next five years received her master's and doctoral degrees from Stanford University.

A life-changing moment came at Stanford when, as a teaching assistant, she first stood before a class of undergraduates. "I felt like a completely different person at that moment," she says. "I realized, this is where I belong. This is what I'm supposed to be doing—leading a class and bringing out the best in students." That realization would reshape her career.

At Oxford University, Connie worked for two years in the legendary Bodleian Library, tracing the ways Shakespeare's plays reflect his early years as a teacher in Stratford-upon-Avon, when children were well-schooled in classical rhetoric. At Yale University, Baldwin would teach again, as an instructor and then assistant professor in the English department. "I have always loved teaching about writing," she says. "I love to help bright young people say what they want to tell the world."

Medical science entered her life in 1978. Connie was in Texas with her husband, a molecular biologist, as well as with a baby and a toddler, when she took a job as a part-time editor and research coordinator for twenty faculty of different disciplines who were studying the biochemistry of schizophrenia at the University of Texas Medical Branch (UTMB) in Galveston. She edited many papers and wrote many grants, learning essential lessons for her future career. As for her shift in academic focus away from Renaissance England, Baldwin says, "You plan things, and then life happens." A glut of baby boomers was vying for too few academic jobs.

At Galveston, teaching others to write well about science became Dr. Baldwin's goal. "Science writing is often murky, and reading much of it is like struggling through a bog," she says. Starting as a research instructor at UTMB, she would teach scientists how to present complex ideas and issues in a language others can understand.

Dr. Baldwin's work as director of the Pediatric Research Office and chair of UTMB's Faculty Development Committee was a critical step upward. With support from a large institutional Robert Wood Johnson Foundation grant (for which she wrote), she developed workshops that taught UTMB's faculty the skills they needed to advance their careers.

As the nation's interconnective technology developed, Baldwin recognized the considerable potential for distance education for health professionals. In 1997, she joined a newly formed consortium of Gulf Coast medical institutions as they entered the expanding world of online education. Teletechnology outreach expanded under Baldwin's leadership into rural Texas, with a three-year project funded by the Health Resources and Services Administration (HRSA) to develop community preceptors' skills in using computers to teach from a distance. The goal was to help healthcare professionals in rural communities educate medical students in the skills of primary care.

Meanwhile, Dr. Baldwin started teaching faculty development workshops on scientific writing at universities all over the country. Every year from 1990–2010, she gave workshops on "Writing Successful Research Grants" and "Nuts and Bolts of Scientific Writing" at professional development conferences of the Association of American Medical Colleges (AAMC) Women in Medicine program. "That adds up to over one thousand aspiring women with writing in their futures," says Baldwin, proudly.

In the early 1990s, a conversation with a UTMB colleague led Baldwin into the national world of academic pediatrics. Professor Harold Levine, a pediatric educator, came to her office one day and said, "I think I can help you to be more successful in your career. I have a plan, and it begins with your curriculum vitae. People who read it must understand what you do. You have to rewrite it."

Connie Baldwin listened. After all, Dr. Levine was a national leader in the AAMC. His plan was this: together he and Baldwin would design a series of joint workshops on educational topics to present at annual meetings of their professional organization, the Academic Pediatric Association (APA). "We can learn together, have fun, and build your credentials as an educator," he pointed out.

Harold Levine was right. His plan would transform both of their careers. In the early 1990s, he introduced Connie to key members of the APA's Education Committee who were starting a major project: revising the curriculum standards for pediatric residency programs at medical schools across the country, some two hundred in all. An editor was needed, and Baldwin volunteered.

"I became part of that core team of senior educators who developed comprehensive goals and objectives for all pediatric residency programs. And these wonderful pediatricians became my closest friends and colleagues," Dr. Baldwin says. The 1996 draft of the *Educational Guidelines for Pediatric Residency* included long lists of goals and objectives in a three-ring binder. Later, the team transformed it, with help from the Josiah Macy Jr. Foundation, into a website loaded with interactive curriculum-building tools. Between 1995 and 2007, the team gave fourteen national workshops on the educational guidelines to get input from residency program directors and teach them how to use these tools.

Because of this visibility, Baldwin was elected chair of APA's Education Committee in 2003. She encouraged the development of the APA's faculty development mission and in 2006 became founding director of the APA Educational Scholars Program (ESP), created for pediatrics faculty whose careers focus on education. Dr. Baldwin considers the ESP to be the most important achievement of her career. Over three years, scholars earn a Certificate of Excellence by attending interactive sessions, engaging in self-directed learning activities, and completing a mentored project with a peer-reviewed scholarly product. To date, 172 scholars have been enrolled and 112 scholars have graduated, with others in the pipeline. In 2016, on its tenth anniversary, the ESP won the prestigious APA Teaching Program Award.

"My work with APA, prompted by Harold Levine, put me on the national scene," Dr. Baldwin says. "Without a medical degree, I became a respected educational expert, valued for having skills—different from those of a clinician—that could benefit my students and colleagues."

Dr. Baldwin was meeting with the *Educational Guidelines* advisory board in Washington, DC, when Dr. Elizabeth McAnarney, then chair of pediatrics at the University of Rochester, saw her in action. Recognizing Baldwin's skill as a group leader, she saw that this was a woman who could enrich the culture of the University of Rochester Department of Pediatrics faculty with her skills in educational scholarship and scientific writing.

Since her arrival in Rochester in 2005, Dr. Baldwin has offered faculty development and grant-writing workshops within the department and across the medical center. She developed a unique scientific writing course for the graduate program that targets pairs of mentors and mentees, who learn together about writing and reviewing articles and grant proposals.

Connie Baldwin credits pioneering feminist Betty Friedan for jolting her out of the earlier, self-limiting mindset of women in her youth. She realized she could aspire to many things as a teacher, unconfined by the walls of a high school classroom. When asked about gender discrimination, she says she has faced only one significant career barrier: not being a physician. "I've been able to bypass all the others, and even that one," she says, "because rather than being part of the competition, I use my gifts to help others succeed. That has always opened doors for me."

"I feel privileged to be working with brilliant people," Dr. Baldwin says, from her sunny, plant-filled office in UR's Saunders Research Building. "I'm here to help them, and they're the ones who are changing the world."

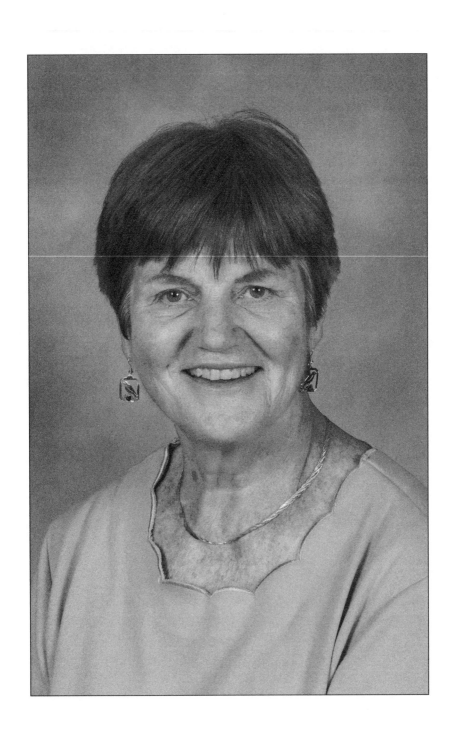

Chapter Four

MARILYN R. BROWN, MD

Dr. Marilyn Brown made her mark as a young pediatrician with her ground-breaking work in nutrition done at the Genesee Hospital (TGH) during the late 1960s. In those days, there was little hope for children whose illness prevented them from absorbing enough nourishment from their food. Without adequate nutrition, the children failed to thrive; some died.

Dr. Brown's work in initiating a potentially life-saving intravenous feeding program for both children and adults was a Rochester "first." "We knew that hospitals in other cities were beginning to develop such programs," she says. "One day, one of our pediatric residents challenged me, asking 'Why don't you start one?'" She did.

Brown enlisted pediatric surgeon Dr. Thomas Putnam in the cause of expanding UR's pediatric service and its facilities at TGH to include the new intravenous treatment. Together they lobbied hospital management for permission to set up a space where the enriched nutritional solutions could be prepared. Technicians were hired to prepare the solutions, monitor the intravenous lines, and keep them clean. Dr. Putnam identified those among his patients who most needed supplemental nourishment at Strong Memorial, Genesee, and Rochester General hospitals. When all was ready, the first were brought in for treatment. "We had wonderful results," Dr. Brown says.

Dr. Brown expanded her expertise in parenteral nutrition therapy and moved across the city to the University of Rochester Medical Center when the pediatric service at TGH ended. There she continued her research on issues related to nutrition, including childhood obesity, and began teaching others, as she does today.

Over the years, Dr. Brown also became involved in medicine within the greater community. She was elected president of the Monroe County Medical Society in 1968 and in 2001 she was elected president of the Rochester Academy of Medicine. In 2013 she was awarded the Academy's prestigious Albert J. Kaiser Medal.

Marilyn du Vigneaud was born in Washington, DC, into a culture extraordinarily rich in science and medicine; her father, Vincent du Vigneaud, was chair of biochemistry at George Washington University at the time. When Marilyn was three, Dr. du Vigneaud became chair of biochemistry at Cornell University Medical College (CUMC) and the family moved to Scarsdale, New York, to be closer to CUMC in Manhattan.

Idyllic summers were spent at the family summer home in Sheffield, Massachusetts. The du Vigneauds' home was built next to that of close friend, Dr. Janet Travell, a pioneer in myofascial pain who later became White House physician for Presidents John F. Kennedy and Lyndon B. Johnson. Science and medicine continued to be staples of conversation around the table.

After graduating from Scarsdale High School in Scarsdale, New York, Marilyn moved north to Ithaca and began her freshman year at Cornell University. Academically her college career was not a straight shot; she sampled both physics and psychology before deciding on medicine. (In 1955, a distraction for the young undergraduate arrived in the form of dramatic family news: Her father had just been awarded the Nobel Prize in Chemistry for the first synthesis of two polypeptide hormones, oxytocin and vasopressin.) A Phi Beta Kappa key came along with Marilyn's Cornell diploma.

In 1957, the new graduate moved to New York City and entered CUMC. Summers during those years were spent doing research at Woods Hole, Massachusetts; La Jolla in California; Boston; and Ithaca. A major change in course—and a very happy one—occurred at the end of her third year at CUMC: Marilyn du Vigneaud married Barry Brown, a law student she had met at Cornell. Barry had a new job with a law firm in Rochester, New York. There, once settled, Marilyn would continue working toward her medical degree at UR.

After completing her remaining course work at UR, including third- and fourth-year psychiatry required by its chairman, Dr. John Romano, Marilyn received her medical degree in 1962. (During her fifth year of medical school, time which focused on research, she gave birth to the Browns' first child, Bruce.) Her link to Genesee Hospital also began that year with her mixed medicine-pediatric internship, later completing pediatrics at Strong Memorial Hospital (SMH).

The birth of the Browns' second child, Gina, in 1965 called for an eight-month break. No jobs were open in pediatrics when she was ready to return, so she clerked briefly at Sibley's, Rochester's iconic downtown department store. In 1966, a position opened at the medical center and Dr. Brown returned to work as a laboratory assistant in virology to Dr. J. B. Hanshaw, with whom she worked for a year on cytomegalovirus.

In 1967, Dr. Brown became a fellow in gastroenterology (adult), researching antibodies related to autoimmune liver disease. The year 1968 was notable: It was marked by the birth of the Browns' third child, Jill, and Dr. Brown began helping develop pediatric gastroenterology at Genesee Hospital, starting her lab there in 1970. She asked a New York City blood bank to send her an Australian antibody and began testing it. It proved to be the antibody for Hepatitis B, and work started flowing into her lab. Shortly afterward, a similar program was begun at Strong Memorial Hospital.

In the early 1970s, Drs. Brown and Putnam initiated the life-saving intravenous nutrition program; Brown's answer to the pediatric resident's challenge: "Why don't you start a program here?" A few years later, Dr. David Smith, the chair of pediatrics, made the controversial decision to close UR support for the pediatrics program at TGH and Marilyn joined other faculty in returning to Strong Memorial Hospital.

At her new base back at the University of Rochester Medical Center, Marilyn worked with the new chief of pediatric gastroenterology, Dr. William Klish, who had been hired from Houston by Dr. Smith. "Dr. Klish was a wonderful person," she recalls, "and really grew the program." Dr. Brown initiated a nutrition support program at SMH, and worked throughout the hospital on nutrition issues, including as director of a weight-control clinic for children and adolescents. Her interest in obesity led to work in the Clinical Research Center with senior scientist Dr. Gilbert Forbes and to the obesity clinic she managed until 1989.

Highlighting her interest in intravenous nutrition, Brown worked with Dr. Harvey Cohen, hematologist/oncologist, to find the cause of muscle weakness in her patients being treated at home. Her paper "Proximal Muscle Weakness and Selenium Deficiency Associated with Long-Term Parenteral Nutrition" was published in 1986.

With Dr. Klish's return to Houston in 1982, the pace of activity within the pediatric GI division slowed and Dr. Brown turned her attention to other activities. She became involved with the Rochester Pediatric Society, the Monroe County Medical Society, and the Rochester Academy of Medicine, eventually serving as president of all three organizations. In 1986, as health-care costs became a high-profile public issue, Dr. Brown joined the board of the Monroe Plan, a Medicaid-managed care organization on whose board she still serves. She was a member of the UR Faculty Senate for twelve years, including six years on the Executive Committee.

In 2000, Buffalo physician Dr. Thomas Rossi joined the GI team of Dr. Tracie Miller and Dr. Brown. Drs. Rossi and Brown began a pediatric gastroenterology fellowship program in 2004. "Tom and I worked hard developing and supporting our first fellows—and I still have the privilege of working within our division with my longtime colleague," says Dr. Brown.

Always innovative, Dr. Brown has reactivated aspects of her early work in nutrition supplementation. Under the leadership of Dr. Lawrence Saubermann, she started a new clinic—Pediatric Advanced Nutrition Support (PANS)—which supports children with tubes for gastrostomy, jejunostomy, or both, or with intravenous lines for nutrition supplementation. "Pediatric GI has grown and improved," she says, with satisfaction. "We have four fantastic young women physicians now. We are at a high, and still growing."

Dr. Brown has held several leadership roles at the UR Medical Center, including director or co-director of nutrition support services at SMH. Currently she directs the education program in gastroenterology/nutrition for medical students and residents.

As she looks back over the early years of her career, Dr. Brown notes an anomaly: "During most of my ten years at Genesee Hospital," she says, "I was essentially working alone. I had freedom there to do things I wanted to do. That was very exciting, phenomenal." At the same time, she says, she really never had a mentor, nor did she have many women colleagues to talk with—one in medicine, a few in pediatrics, one in surgery, five in the medical school at UR.

Mentors *are* important, though, and Dr. Brown advises young women coming into the profession to work at developing strong relationships with faculty who share their professional interests. She herself has honored in a very special way the woman who helped her, longtime department chair Elizabeth McAnarney. As president of the Rochester Pediatric Society, a division of the Rochester Academy of Medicine, Dr. Brown energized colleagues to establish an annual pediatric grand rounds lectureship in Dr. McAnarney's name, a program now seventeen years old.

If finding appropriate mentors is important, so is a continuing process of self-assessment, Dr. Brown says. What do you want to do with your life? Do you have the drive to be single-minded about career advancement? "Devotion to work is good," she says, and so is a life that includes other dimensions, including ties to the greater community.

For many years an avid squash and tennis player and a horseback rider, Dr. Brown has found a new interest: her involvement with Rochester's Garth Fagan dance company. Twenty years ago, she designed and had built a retirement home for herself and husband Barry, close to the landmark farmhouse near Mendon Ponds Park where they lived for more than thirty years. She says she will always remember early morning hours caring for her horses there before a long day at the hospital.

As important as her honors—the prestigious Kaiser medal, an Award of Merit from the Rochester Academy of Medicine, a Ruth A. Lawrence Faculty Service Award, and listings in *Best Doctors in America* and *Cambridge Who's Who*—Dr. Brown says her proudest achievements are her three children and five grandchildren.

In summary, Dr. Brown says, "I have thoroughly enjoyed my work and my interactions with patients, families, nurses, medical students, residents, and faculty." The past twelve years have brought Dr. Brown a special pleasure, as she works with young doctors in the fellowship program whose design and content she helped shape.

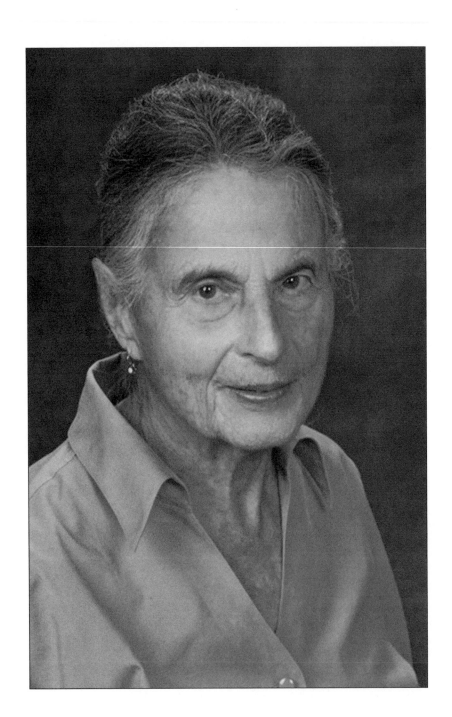

Chapter Five

CENIE C. CAFARELLI, MD

Dr. Cenie Cafarelli can't say how many thousands of children she has taken care of during the course of her forty-two-year career. She's pleased, but never surprised, each time she's greeted at the grocery store or post office by a former patient, or by the mother of a former patient. After all, that's what her career has been all about: taking care of children.

". . . and their families," Dr. Cafarelli adds, with emphasis. That was the critical element that drew her to pediatrics. "Originally, I planned to specialize in family medicine. Of course, I soon realized that treating children would connect me with their families, too." As a pediatrician, she would be involved in a complex world that includes patient, parents, and siblings, sometimes all in her office together.

Dr. Cafarelli was one of the first physicians in Rochester chosen to mentor the pioneering nurses who, in the 1960s, became nurse practitioners, the second such cadre in the nation. For most of her career, though, she has been a beloved private practitioner as well as a preceptor for medical students.

Dr. Cafarelli is a senior member of the American Academy of Pediatrics, Monroe County Medical Society, and the Rochester Academy of Medicine.

As the only child of a father who was a physician, it was perhaps inevitable that Cenie would be drawn to medicine. Her father was a military surgeon with the Sixth Armored Division, whose preparation for the Normandy invasion took the family across the US to various military training bases. It was he who encouraged her to consider medical school. This was uncommon parental advice for a woman during the 1950s, when few women considered becoming doctors—and far fewer were accepted, much less welcomed, in medical schools.

As young Cenie passed through one state school district after another, she often learned more about life than what each curriculum offered. Of her two years as a primary student at a rural school in Bradenton, Kentucky, she says "I learned more at that school than at most others, for a simple reason: The students in this small county seat were diverse, and the teachers taught the basics in a shortened school year." Basics indeed. No indoor plumbing at that school, just two outhouses. When spring arrived in March, the school year ended so that students could work with their families on the farms.

By the time Cenie was thirteen, she had lived near military posts in Virginia, Kentucky, Arkansas, and California. Along the way, her future was becoming clear. "I knew I liked science and math," she says. "I was good at both. I was also good with people. It looked like a medical career would not only work for me, but give me joy."

There was a war going during the 1940s, a big one. As World War II exploded, Cenie's father was ordered to Germany with the Sixth Armored Division. Cenie and her mother also moved, back to Westchester County where her mother had roots and her father had family living in the lower Hudson Valley. At high school in Ossining, New York, Cenie reaffirmed her interest in science. (During the school's "Technology Day," she was the only girl to participate.) As a Girl Scout, she traveled after high school to an international encampment in Sweden. Another war-time summer, Cenie and her mother spent several weeks in Colorado, riding horses and exploring the mountains.

In September 1949, Cenie entered Vassar College in nearby Poughkeepsie. She credits those college years with supporting her independent spirit. Three years at Vassar fulfilled admission requirements to Albany Medical College. "At the time, Albany was the smallest medical school in the country," she says. "It was the right choice for me. I wasn't interested in climbing a career ladder, I wanted to do family medicine. At Albany, we felt that our professors supported us and wanted us to succeed." As for gender bias, she says she encountered none.

Dr. Cenie Cafarelli received her medical degree in 1958, and late that summer began her rotating internship at Rochester General Hospital (RGH), where several classmates had led the way. As they had in Albany, Cenie and her mother shared a house, this time on Portland Avenue. The interns' days and nights were split between Rochester General on Portland Avenue, known as "Northside," and its urban component on Troup Street, "Westside."

The work was grueling, Dr. Cafarelli recalls. For a time, she was the only intern in the Emergency Department; when serious cases arrived, she phoned for support from the hospital's experienced doctors. "During the internship, we were on-call for 36 hours followed by 12 hours off," she recalls. "As we worked our way that year through the Emergency Department, Internal Medicine, Obstetrics, and Pediatrics, I learned a tremendous amount of medicine from the variety of patients we treated, the diseases we encountered, and from attending doctors."

When her rotating internship ended, Cenie took a much-needed personal year off, traveling across the country with her mother, visiting family, and returning to places where they had lived. Residency in internal medicine at RGH the next year was followed by a year in Philadelphia, where she was enrolled in the Graduate School of Internal Medicine at the University of Pennsylvania. Since this was strictly an academic program, she had time to explore the Philadelphia area with a hiking group.

Pediatrics as a career choice was beginning to prevail over family medicine, and in 1964 she began her two-year pediatric residency at RGH under pediatrician Dr. Edward Townsend. In the early years of RGH's affiliation with Strong Memorial, Dr. Townsend had volunteered to run this integrated rotation for medical students, a program that included six months of clinical work at Strong Memorial Hospital.

In 1964, Dr. Cafarelli was named an associate resident in pediatrics, with a focus on endocrinology and metabolic disorders at the UR School of Medicine and Dentistry. The Endocrinology and Metabolism Clinic provided comprehensive care for many diverse patients. During the second year of this residency, Dr. Cafarelli worked as a research fellow with Dr. Gilbert Forbes, a distinguished biophysicist and radiation biologist who had worked at Los Alamos and Oxford, and who was now a member of the Department of Pediatrics. Dr. Forbes and a colleague had discovered a new method of determining lean body weight by measuring gamma rays emitted by natural potassium [K]-40. Dr. Cafarelli and others on Forbes's team assessed the body composition and fat-to-muscle ratios of schoolchildren enrolled in the studies.

By 1966, the time had come. The promise of independence in a private practice led Dr. Cafarelli to open her own office. She'd worked with children as a resident and as a researcher, but in private practice she could make taking care of children her first priority. The big question was: Where to establish that practice? Before making her decision, Dr. Cafarelli visited each of the several places where she had lived, researching their social and economic environments. None seemed as propitious as Rochester. Her first office as a solo practitioner was in the Towne House on Mt. Hope Avenue, adjacent to SMH.

A year later, she moved her expanding practice a mile away to Westfall Park and added new supporting staff. A skilled group of like-minded pediatricians provided cross-coverage and after-hours relief. Such teamwork is key, she says: "Every member of an office team, from those at the front desk to those providing follow-up calls and care, are all-important to the success of a medical practice."

In 1968, Dr. Cafarelli had the opportunity to be part of the pioneering nurse practitioner movement. The Baby Boom of the 1950s and '60s exploded just as many medical students were turning to specialty practices and away from general medicine. UR chair of pediatrics Dr. Robert Haggerty worked closely with faculty from the School of Nursing to fast-forward a pediatric nurse practitioner program in Rochester. Dr. Cafarelli helped train one of the first four nurses chosen to initiate the program, which included a four-month academic program, followed by two years providing well-patient care in a pediatrician's office, health care center, or clinic. Nurse practitioners became an integral part of her practice.

After her retirement in 2008, Dr. Cafarelli continued to bring her professional skills to others, as a volunteer pediatrician at St. Joseph's Neighborhood Center and as an attending, without admitting privileges, co-rounding for resident teaching at SMH.

Currently, she is an active volunteer for organizations that work to protect the environment, a cause that has meant much to her for many years. As a board member of the Genesee Land Trust, she chairs its Land Management Committee and she is treasurer of the local chapter of the Sierra Club. A committed environmentalist, she says, "Climate change will continue to be a challenge, as new diseases spread into previously too cold environments and earth's ecosystems are stressed."

In a career that lasted nearly fifty years, Dr. Cafarelli found what she had been looking for: work that had great value and that would bring her joy. ("I also liked being in charge," she says, with a smile.) "Practicing primary care medicine has been very rewarding, with many intellectual challenges. Equally important are the long-term patient relationships that I've developed, including some of three-generation duration."

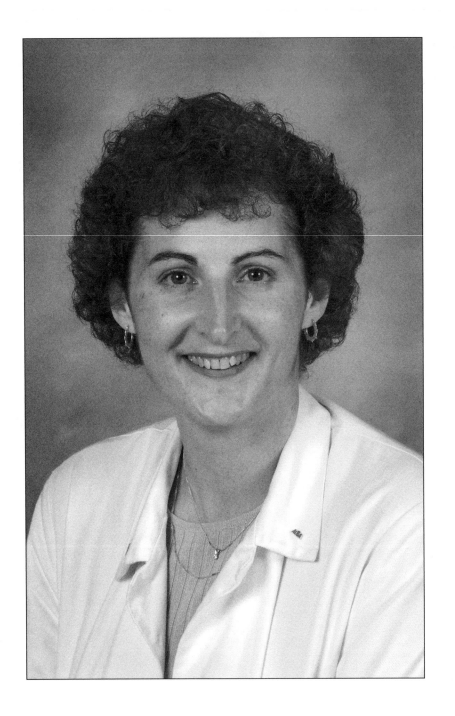

Chapter Six

Mary T. Caserta, MD

Sooner or later, every child gets an infectious disease. Usually it is only a troubling discomfort, an excuse perhaps to sleep late on a school day. Unfortunately, it may leave a disfiguring signature. Tragically, it can even be lethal.

Dr. Mary Caserta clearly remembers having a serious infection, measles, as a child. Whether or not those red spots presaged her future as one of the University of Rochester's leading infectious disease (ID) investigators is a hypothetical question. She is sure, however, that her interest in infectious diseases and public health began early and remains strong.

For more than twenty years, starting in 1991, Dr. Caserta worked in the URMC laboratory of ID specialist Dr. Caroline Breese Hall, known worldwide for her research on Human Herpesvirus-6 (HHV-6) and Respiratory Syncytial Virus (RSV), leading causes of illness in babies and young children. Dr. Hall grounded her young mentee in the basics of translational virology. Now, Dr. Caserta has expanded her early research vision beyond the realm of human herpesviruses and into respiratory viral infections.

Dr. Caserta knows that medical science needs to find ways to understand how viruses can cause severe respiratory disease in young children. In 2011, the URMC was awarded a seven-year contract totaling $35 million from the National Institute of Allergy and Infectious Diseases (NIAID) to fund a Respiratory Pathogens Research Center (RPRC). Dr. Caserta, who contributed to the winning proposal, is now the Center's Pediatric Clinical Core Director and works on two of its primary research programs.

"Mary is one of our research stars," says Dr. Elizabeth McAnarney, emerita chair of the Department of Pediatrics. Dr. Caserta is busier than ever now, engrossed in work that aims to help children—and adults—afflicted by the most common of the world's multitude of viruses.

Mary Caserta's rise to career success is inspiring, and her family story is complex. Her paternal grandfather immigrated to the US around the turn of the twentieth century, settling his family in western Pennsylvania where he worked in the coal mines. Mary's father, one of ten children in that first-generation Italian American family, worked as a factory maintenance man at the Sealtest Ice Cream Company in Buffalo.

Mary's father and three of his siblings were congenitally deaf. Her mother, an orphan, was adopted by an older couple who both died when she was just a teenager. As a result, Mary's mother moved in with her aunt and uncle who also were deaf, as were her cousins. It perhaps was inevitable that Mary's parents would meet at a social club associated with St. Mary's School for the Deaf in Buffalo.

Money was tight in the Caserta household. "Our pediatrician was our household hero," says Mary. "He made house calls, and I remember him saying, 'Well, mother, what's going on here?' We often had to run up a tab, but each spring, my mother would pay the bill from the tax return money. He took good care of us."

Many lessons were learned in that household in Buffalo, and they didn't all come from books. "My parents were good people who worked hard all their lives at jobs they didn't like," says Dr. Caserta. "But they were able to provide opportunities for my brother and me." (Mary's brother is a lawyer, one cousin has a doctoral degree, other cousins are nurse practitioners or have other higher-level degrees.) As for her parents' hopes for the next generation, Mary says, "It was all about getting a good education. After that, you chart your own destiny."

Mary went to the all-girls Buffalo Academy of the Sacred Heart. As graduation approached, so did thoughts of college. "It was so different then," she recalls. "You didn't apply to many schools. I had applied to the University of Buffalo and Syracuse University, when one day a recruiter from Marquette [University] came to Sacred Heart. I went to Milwaukee to visit the university, and loved it. Like Sacred Heart, it was a school with a strong sense of community—plus, they offered me a full academic scholarship." Another incentive was that, since Mary's mother worked for the railroad, she could ride at half-fare between Milwaukee and Buffalo.

At Marquette, Mary's work/study program linked her with a professor in the dental school; she worked as one of his laboratory technicians on studies of blood coagulation. She graduated in 1980 with a clear understanding of where her professional future would be grounded—in medical research—and with a bachelor's degree in science, *summa cum laude*.

Mary entered SUNY Buffalo School of Medicine that September. During her first year, she met her first important clinical mentor, pediatric hematologist/oncologist Dr. Richard Sills. "Rich was wonderful. He took time to see that I got clinical experience. He took me into a surgical suite to watch a C-section delivery, where everything was organized, neat, and timely. Next, he had me watch a vaginal delivery, an experience which completely shocked me. So much noise, so much blood!"

In his laboratory, Dr. Sills was investigating why children with serious infections, such as meningitis, also became anemic. Not only did Mary work in Sills's lab, she was the control in many of his experiments; every day she would have her own blood taken, measured, and analyzed. Eventually, enough data were gathered for a scientific paper on which Mary Caserta's name appears as second author. "At Marquette, I was a 'lab tech,'" Dr. Caserta says. "Working with Rich, I was on the road to becoming a real scientist."

In 1984, Dr. Mary Caserta received her medical degree, *summa cum laude*. Just before graduation, she flew to Thailand, where she worked for several weeks at a refugee camp sponsored by Catholic Relief Services near the Cambodian border. Her previous elective rotation in ID at Rochester General Hospital with Dr. Edward Walsh had prepared her for the trip by reviewing pathogens common in pediatrics. When a refugee child's symptoms suggested a possible central nervous system infection, Mary did her first spinal tap, a procedure which revealed the problem was typhoid. "Those weeks in Thailand gave me a chance to learn a lot about medicine, public health, *and* about myself," she says.

Back in the US, Dr. Caserta spent the next three years at the Children's Hospital of Philadelphia (CHOP) as a resident. CHOP was an exciting place to be for infectious disease specialists. Dr. H. Frederick Clark, professor of pediatrics, would soon have a profound impact on world health with his successful rotavirus vaccine, co-invented during those years with CHOP Infectious Diseases chief Stanley Plotkin, MD and Paul Offit, MD. The vaccine's advent eventually would save hundreds of thousands of children worldwide from severe disease.

Dr. Caserta's next research experience began in Dr. Clark's laboratory, where she infected mice with a virus fresh from the freezer. The question being asked: Would a cold-adapted rotavirus strain produce mild symptoms? As the experiment progressed, it was apparent the vaccine was *not* attenuated and therefore would not be a good candidate to move forward. The result was not failure, of course, but one more carefully documented step along a research pathway. Mary was learning the importance of persistence.

By 1987, Dr. Caserta, newly married, told Dr. Plotkin that she would be leaving CHOP to move to Rochester, New York, with her lawyer husband. "In that case you can work with my friend Caren Hall," he told her, and went on to explain Dr. Hall's game-changing work with RSV. The connection would be transformational. "Caren taught me how to do translational research, work that involved not mice and test tubes, but humans," says Dr. Caserta. Over the next twenty-one years, Hall's knowledge and wisdom would shape her mentee's life in ways both professional and personal.

Mary's UR career began as an instructor and fellow in pediatric infectious diseases and immunology at a time when Dr. Hall was on sabbatical. On Hall's return, she took the exceptional new fellow under her wing. In 1991, under

Hall's guidance, Dr. Caserta began the research that would dominate her career: studying the clinical characteristics of HHV-6 and, most recently, other respiratory pathogens that sicken and sometimes kill thousands of children each year.

The recent research successes of UR faculty Drs. David Topham, Ann Falsey, Caserta, and others resulted in the breakthrough NIAID contract to establish UR's Respiratory Pathogens Research Center. As director of the center's Pediatric Clinical Core, Dr. Caserta is involved in two important ventures with Drs. Edward Walsh and Gloria Pryhuber. The first is an investigation of how RSV infection can cause severe disease in previously well, full-term newborns. The second major thrust explores how repeated respiratory infections in both preterm and full-term newborns can cause respiratory disease in later childhood, as investigators examine the infections' effects on the microbiome and developing immune system.

Dr. Caserta also works with Thomas O'Connor, PhD, and Jan Moynihan, PhD, colleagues in Psychiatry, who are studying how psychosocial stress impacts pregnancy and the child's developing immune system, susceptibility to infectious diseases, and overall health.

A teacher as well as a researcher, Dr. Caserta's effectiveness is proven by multiple awards, including the Outstanding Hospital Faculty Teaching Award, the Medicine/Pediatrics Award for Teaching Excellence, the Faculty Teaching Award in Pediatrics for third-year medical students, and the Pediatric Morning Report Teaching Award, the latter three years in a row.

Dr. Caserta is a member of several national advisory health councils and research review committees, most often for Pediatric Academic Societies; in 2014 she co-chaired the NAIAD workshop on Roseola-viruses.

Much of her early success, Dr. Caserta says, is due to her mentor, Dr. Hall. "Caren supported me in so many ways, including one of the most essential, helping me find funding," she says.

That help could also take a personal turn. A day came when Caserta's career trajectory was challenged by a man in higher authority. Devastated, she turned for counsel to Dr. Hall, who asked: "What do you want to do with your life?" Mary responded, "I really think I can make a contribution in research." Championed by Dr. Hall, Mary Caserta decided to stay the course at URMC, and flourished.

A true crisis shadowed Dr. Caserta's early years in Rochester. Her first pregnancy ended tragically with the death of twins. During those difficult days, Dr. Hall helped see her through. When a second—and ultimately successful—pregnancy required thirty weeks of bed rest, Mary again had Dr. Hall's support. ("I would have stood on my head for thirty weeks to save that baby," she says.) Two years later, when Mary approached Dr. Hall about the possibility of a third pregnancy, Hall smiled and suggested she use the "Twenty-Year Rule." "What will impact your life more significantly," she asked. "A series of experiments in the lab, or a decision to expand your family?" The children of this third pregnancy (again twins) are now both college graduates.

Young women coming into medicine who are concerned about combining career and family may learn from Dr. Caserta's experience as a busy researcher and mother of three children. "It's easier now than it was years ago," she says, "but still a challenge. It's a balancing act that is doable, if you're not doing it alone. Get help and a good partner. My husband really went the extra mile. He's done a lot of the heavy lifting. And, unlike me, he never was late for a soccer practice."

Throughout her career, Mary Caserta has focused on the joys of working with children. "I love their innocence and the potential for good health outcomes. And I love their resilience. I think my brother and I benefitted from a degree of benign neglect from our parents that fostered resilience. I believe that has benefitted me very well."

Dr. Mary Caserta's final words of advice for those entering the profession:

- Determine where you can make your best contribution.
- Remember, perseverance is the key to success.
- Follow Dr. Hall's "Twenty-Year Rule": When faced with a significant career decision, ask yourself this question: What will make the most important impact in my life twenty years from now?

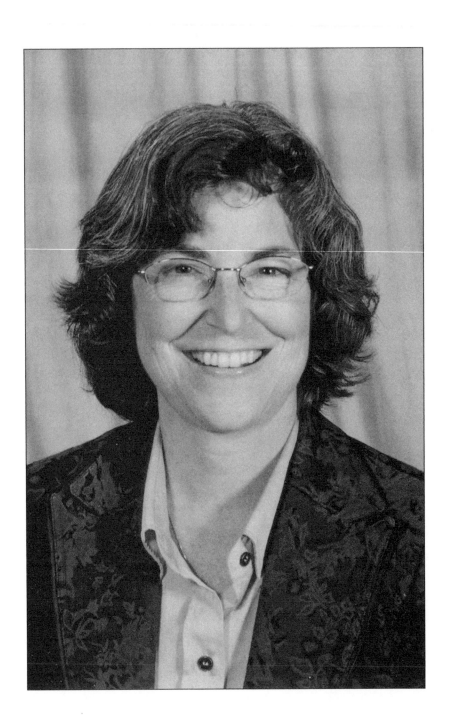

Chapter Seven

Patricia R. Chess, MD

Patricia R. Chess, a neonatologist, biomedical scientist, and distinguished teacher and mentor, is partnering with UR River Campus biomedical engineers to design and create twenty-first-century tools to save premature infants struggling with respiratory crises, as well as those born with specific physical anomalies. This new work marks a career turn for Dr. Chess, who has been on the list of Best Doctors in America since 2004.

Recently Chess and her team introduced their latest achievement: a respiratory monitor so sensitive that it registers tiny changes in chest wall movements, as small as 5 percent, occurring in the lungs of critically ill babies being supported on ventilators that breathe four hundred to nine hundred times a minute. The monitor's alarm alerts Neonatal Intensive Care Unit (NICU) staff to an urgent problem. No previous monitor is as exquisitely calibrated. Earlier, the Chess team created and patented a three-dimensional patch to support babies born with a diaphragmatic hernia, a congenital disorder that can allow abdominal organs to intrude into the chest cavity where they inhibit lung function.

Helping design and bringing into medical practice these devices is only one facet of Chess's work, which continues to be teaching and working with the most compromised of the NICU's infants. Dr. Chess says her greatest source of professional pride is her success in bringing the pediatric heart-lung bypass capability called Extra-Corporeal Membrane Oxygenation (ECMO) to Rochester. She first learned about ECMO at Columbia University where she saw how it could save the lives of sickly babies with a reversible breathing problem. Before 1998, babies with similar problems in Rochester were flown to other centers where the technology—and the skills required to use it—was available; tragically, some babies died en route. "I really fought for this," she says. "I said, 'I'm not staying if we don't get ECMO." Dr. Chess is the medical director of ECMO at URMC, recently one of sixteen medical centers whose program received "Gold Standard" certification from the national Extracorporeal Life Support Organization.

The paths to career success and satisfaction are many and varied. Now near the apex of her career, Dr. Chess's path began in the URMC laboratory of Jacob Finkelstein, PhD, and later with Robert Notter MD, PhD. During the early 1980s, Drs. Finkelstein and Notter and their group of pulmonary biomedical scientists forged revolutionary advances in neonatal lung research, including using surfactant extracted from calves' lungs to treat premature infants with lung insufficiency who were failing from acute respiratory distress. Dr. Chess worked with the neonatal lung laboratory group for fifteen years, helping refine respiratory support, response to injury, and the complex lipoprotein surfactant treatment. Their advances had national impact. "For years, we thought we were fortunate if we could save infants born at twenty-eight weeks. Now we're having success at twenty-three weeks," she says.

A Rochesterian through and through, Dr. Chess is the sixth of seven children born to a six-generation Rochester family. "I knew as early as fourth grade that I wanted a career that would enable me to help children and teach others," she says. This early decision worried her Catholic parents, who at that time favored a more traditional role for their girls. "They thought I was an 'aberration,' but eventually, they were proud of me," she says, with a smile, gesturing to the four handsome young adults whose photographs grace her office, the children from her thirty-year marriage to radiologist Dr. Mitchell Chess. All four offspring are UR graduates.

After graduating as valedictorian from Rochester's Cardinal Mooney High School, Patty worked to pay her way through Colgate University, graduating with a double-major in mathematics and chemistry. She understood that she had a calling for a career in science, but could she be both a doctor and a mother; have both a husband and a medical career? As the first in her family to pursue a career in medicine, she was startled to be told at one medical school interview: "You can't be a good doctor and a good mother." She bristled at the advice and ignored that application. A professor at Colgate had a more positive suggestion. "You must talk to Ruth Lawrence at the University of Rochester," the friend said, and she described the near-legendary UR pediatrician who had both a sterling career *and* a family, including nine children. During a month of independent study as a child life specialist at URMC, Patty met with Dr. Lawrence; their conversation finalized her decision to apply to medical school.

In life, obstacles sooner or later seem to arise, blocking our course, sometimes when we are least equipped to meet them. Patty learned this soon after making the decision to apply to medical school. Her academic record at Colgate was splendid—straight A's, research experience, and the right extra-curricular achievements. But, with money tight, she had applied to only three medical schools, all of the interviews for which were scheduled for the same week. That timing couldn't have been worse. Her beloved mother, her "kindred spirit," had just been diagnosed with cancer and the young graduate was badly shaken emotionally. She was wait-listed at all three schools—and she had no Plan B. (A life lesson learned, she says: "Always have a Plan B.")

Undeterred, Patty went to work teaching in a chemistry lab at Colgate, banking her paychecks. At the end of the year, she had saved enough to apply to ten medical schools. With a number of options this time around, she chose Columbia University College of Physicians and Surgeons, where she won honors in pediatrics in 1988 and chose her specialty, neonatology.

At Columbia, she also met another prize: medical student Mitchell Chess, who would become her husband. "I knew I wanted a husband, not just a paycheck," she says. "[Mitchell] was one of the brightest men I'd ever met, and one of the funniest and kindest." It was the latter quality that won her. As her mother's health failed and death approached, Patty felt alone and bereft in Manhattan. Mitchell came to her and said, "You need a friend now. I'm going to be that friend." He made sure she headed back to Rochester immediately and took her to the train heading upstate; she arrived home just hours before her mother died. "That's the kind of person you want to be with you for the rest of your life," she says. She urges other young people to look for the same qualities in a life partner.

Patty and Mitchell married while they were in medical school and looked forward to beginning what both hoped would become the kind of big, comfortable family that Patty was used to. Then the unthinkable happened—the young couple's first child died shortly after birth of severe congenital abnormalities. "We were both devastated," she says. "I thought, there's no way now I can do pediatrics. How can I possibly do that?" One day, not long after the tragedy, Patty was assigned to a family whose infant was dying. "I remember going into a hospital restroom and sobbing, just sobbing, thinking this was impossible, I can't do this," she recalls. Then, somehow, in that room she realized she was the perfect person to help this mother. She'd been through the pain and, with help, had come out the other side.

Over the following months, the young doctor's grief ebbed, and exactly a year to the day later, when Patty was an intern, baby Rachel was born, healthy and beautiful. Laura arrived on the scene when her mother was a pediatric chief resident; Daniel when she was a neonatal fellow; and Stephen when she was a junior faculty member. Two weeks after Stephen was born, his mother submitted her first funded National Institutes of Health (NIH) grant.

The Drs. Chess arrived in Rochester in 1988, Patty as a pediatric intern, Mitchell as a radiology resident. In 2009, Patty Chess was chosen to direct the neonatology fellowship training program. Four years later she was picked to oversee all pediatric subspecialty fellowship training programs and in 2014, she became vice chair of education for pediatrics. In 2015 she became chair of the national Organization of Neonatology Training Program Directors. "I like to keep busy!" she says, with a smile.

All this leads one to ask: How can all this be accomplished? A mentor who shares your professional interest is an asset beyond price. Dr. Chess says she's had many significant mentors. We've seen how Ruth Lawrence influenced the young student to choose pediatrics as her profession; over the years, she has continued to be a wise and supportive presence. Lung biology researcher Jack Finkelstein became an important mentor during Dr. Chess's neonatology fellowship years. While the lab work was focused on type-2 epithelial cells, an important focus of Chess's early work, Dr. Finkelstein's influence went far beyond the benchwork. "He was a wise ear," she says. "It's because he showed me the strength of the neonatology program that I stayed here." Dr. Elizabeth McAnarney, chair of pediatrics (now emerita chair), is another mentor, "one who puts things into a unique personal and professional perspective."

As a mentor herself, Dr. Chess reaps praise from her own mentees. Kristin Scheible, MD, a former UR fellow and current neonatology faculty member, associate director of the neonatal ECMO program and physician scientist, is one of many who have learned from her. "Dr. Chess was always patient with us residents as we navigated the great unknowns in the NICU: how to assess and present patients, how to talk to parents and nurses, how to read an X-ray. She is the 'go-to' provider for the most acute and complicated patients, identifying clinical learning opportunities for us and ensuring that her trainees are present for all management decisions.

"All the fellows would turn to Patty when we were trying to figure out our best career path, even before she was named the program's director. Because she took time to get to know us, she could help us integrate all the pieces into our own personal career plan, one that balances competing agendas—one that will make us happy."

Patty Chess says her greatest personal pride is in the family's four children: all UR graduates; Rachel, who teaches physics and biology in the Boston Public School district; Laura, a biomedical engineer working in Boston; Daniel, a brain and cognitive development specialist working as a therapist in Portland,

Oregon; and Stephen, working in optical engineering in New Hampshire. "As the children were growing, I insisted on three things," she says. "They had to do something musical, something athletic, and something for the community." Her goal for them all: Be happy—and leave the world a better place.

Dr. Chess has some powerful advice for young people: First, choose your life partner wisely. Next, be flexible—and always have a Plan B. Make being organized a lifelong practice. When challenged with multiple choices, always ask yourself what is important to *you*. Learn to say "no" (politely, as in, "I'll have to think about that"). Examine what it takes to be respected within your institution. Learn how to advance up the career ladder in an appropriate way, supporting those junior to you. Always continue learning; don't stagnate. (Dr. Chess admits she was fortunate to have an ace in the hole when it was needed: her large, supportive family. Last year the family's Thanksgiving gathering topped out at fifty.)

Finally, "take time for yourself," says this woman who has done just that, throughout a long and successful career. Every week she and her husband take time out for ballroom dancing!

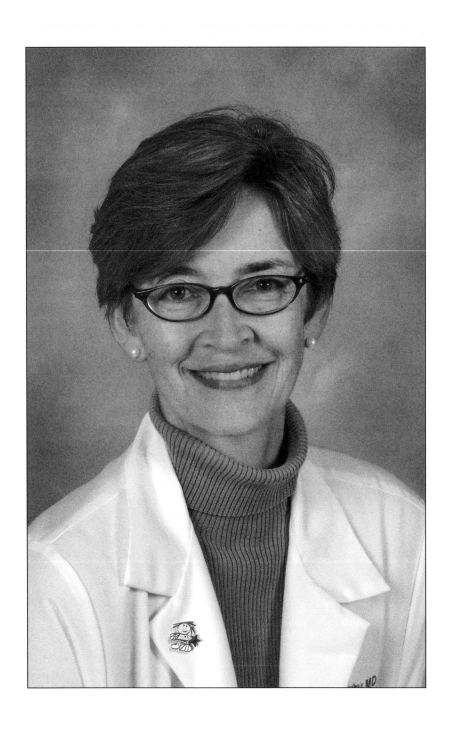

Chapter Eight

CYNTHIA CHRISTY, MD

For a new doctor, it's often life, as much as what happens in the medical school classroom, that shapes a profession. One of Dr. Cynthia Christy's most powerful learning experiences unfolded during her first years of residency at the University of Kentucky. Here was an environment far different from that of New England, where she had spent eight years of undergraduate education and medical training. "The poverty I saw in Kentucky, especially among the families living in the mountains, was eye-opening. Our clinics were full of very sick people with complex and fascinating problems," she recalls.

Today, Dr. Christy, a pediatric infectious disease (ID) specialist, is among the UR Department of Pediatrics faculty helping teach young doctors how to become even better doctors. That she is good at the job is clear: three classes of medical students and residents have honored her with Outstanding Faculty Teaching Awards. As they enter the real world of medicine, these doctors will be taking on many of the same challenges that Dr. Christy met when her career began. The long chain of learning/teaching/outreach will continue.

At Jackson College, which was then Tufts University's college for women, Cynthia on a whim took a music course that changed her life. Also enrolled in "Music 8" was a young pre-med student from Maine, Ralph Manchester; after many walks back and forth to class, the young couple became engaged. (The young man is now Dr. Ralph Manchester, vice provost of the University of Rochester, director of University Health, and professor of medicine.)

After graduating from Tufts in 1975, Cynthia spent six months at the University of Maryland Medical School before joining her fiancé at the University of Vermont College of Medicine (UVM). "The summer before I entered UVM, I worked as a lifeguard at a camp in Maine," she says. "I taught the class with the youngest kids, and I loved working with them. There was lots of laughing." That sun-filled summer, she thinks, was the spark that eventually led her to pediatrics.

Cynthia's favorite teacher at UVM was ID specialist Dr. Carol Phillips. "Women were a minority in medical school in those days. To get ahead, I had to work hard," she recalls. Cynthia and Ralph successfully "couples-matched" for their residency training at the University of Kentucky in Lexington and left for the South after their graduation from UVM in 1979.

At Kentucky, Dr. Christy was influenced by one of the "great women of pediatrics," Dr. Jacqueline Noonan, a former UVM medical student, then chair of the Department of Pediatrics at Kentucky. Cynthia focused on her pediatric residency. She learned a lot while working in Noonan's department, and she took away a few life lessons, as well. From Dr. Noonan she learned the importance of the word "compromise." Noonan told her residents, "Even though you may think you can do everything in your career and in your personal life, you probably can't. Learn the value of compromise." If a resident confided that he or she was stressed, unhappy at work, Noonan would withhold sympathy, suggesting instead that the student reevaluate the situation, looking perhaps for a different career focus, one where he or she would find the kind of satisfaction that Noonan had in cardiology.

Dr. Christy brought her family to Rochester during the summer of 1983, Ralph as an internist in Medicine and Cynthia as an instructor with a two-year National Institutes of Health fellowship in pediatric infectious disease and immunology; the fellowship would be renewed two years later.

When no faculty position was open in Pediatrics on Crittenden Boulevard, she moved to Rochester General Hospital as an attending physician and found herself with a vibrant group of young new colleagues. Now, nearly three decades later, half of Dr. Christy's time is devoted to teaching. In addition, she manages the care of babies and children with infections at both Golisano Children's Hospital and RGH. "I wear many hats, and I love it!" Dr. Christy says.

Dr. Christy's interest in ID research is ongoing, although active participation is limited now by her teaching, administrative, and clinical duties. Over the past fifteen years she has participated in studies of tuberculosis screening for inner city children and on the effect of the influenza vaccine in children with asthma. At healthcare meetings, she has presented on two "super bugs," oxacillin-resistant *Staphylococcus aureus* (ORSA) and methicillin-resistant *Staphylococcus aureus* (MRSA), and their infections in children; urinary tract infections; H1N1 influenza; fever of unknown origin; meningitis; and measles.

Dr. Christy is active within her profession both nationally and locally. A fellow of the American Academy of Pediatrics and of the Infectious Disease Society of America, she is also active as a medical educator in the Council on Medical Student Education in Pediatrics (COMSEP). With other COMSEP members, she is active in educational research efforts, including ways to encourage community pediatricians to use their offices as teaching environments.

Dr. Christy's job is a big one, with many responsibilities—including raising three children. She says that finding the right balance is what has made it work for her—and that includes having energy and a very helpful husband. "Raising kids is a team sport! That's the scaffolding that holds it all together," she says.

"There will be low spots in your career," she counsels young people coming into the profession. "The workplace can be warm and collegial, but it is not a family." At a low point in her own career and facing a painful interpersonal challenge, she was helped by department chair Dr. Elizabeth McAnarney. During that period of introspection, Dr. Christy says she gained self-knowledge that since has been very useful.

One of the joys of Cynthia Christy's career is her involvement with students. "I love being with young people. They're so bright, so energetic, so thirsty for knowledge," she says. "Every year I meet a new group, and I learn with them. As a medical educator, if I can make a lifelong impact on at least one student each year, I'll consider my work a success."

Here are three tips from a physician who knows her work—and loves it.

- Spend time talking with friends who are supportive.
- Develop good communication lines with faculty.
- Find your niche—and enjoy it!

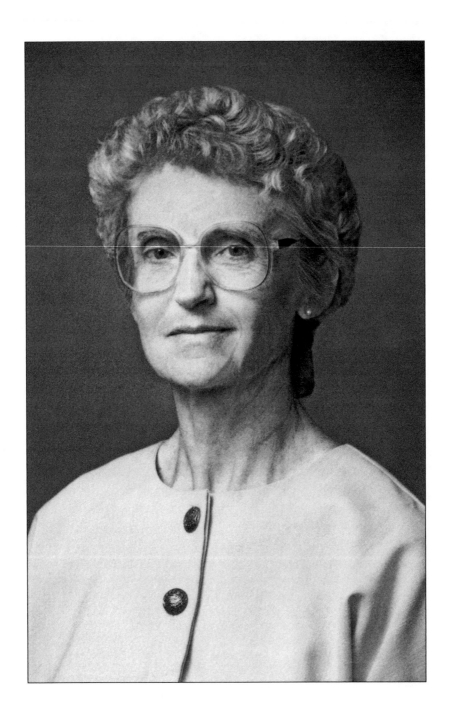

Chapter Nine

Margaret T. Colgan, MD (1928–2018)[1]

Dr. Margaret Colgan, a revered professor of pediatrics and longtime chief of the Pediatric Residency Program at the University of Rochester, lived in retirement in Annapolis, Maryland, until her death in 2018. "Meg was a fast-moving will-o'-the-wisp," says Peggy McFarlane Rickman, coordinator of the Pediatric Residency Program during the 1980s and early '90s. "She was down to earth, funny, and a joy to be around. Her open-door policy made her very accessible to both faculty and residents. She had a special gift—as a mother of five with a disabled child, she really knew how to relate to worried parents."

"She was magical," agrees Marilyn Brown, MD, professor of pediatrics, who worked with Dr. Colgan throughout their early careers. "Everyone loved her. Not only was she an excellent clinical teacher, she had a very special way of interacting with residents. I remember one young man in academic trouble who went into Meg's office wearing a very worried look. He came out smiling. I wondered at the time how she learned that skill."

Dr. Colgan was the first woman to serve as president of the Rochester Academy of Medicine. Over the course of her distinguished career she held key roles at three Rochester hospitals; as director of both pediatric education and the pediatric clinic at Rochester General Hospital; Pediatrician-in-Chief at the Genesee Hospital; and director of the Pediatric Residency Program and the Ambulatory Pediatric Clinic at Strong Memorial Hospital.

Her talents as a teacher and medical educator in general pediatrics were recognized in 1992 when she was awarded the University's Gold Medal Award honoring her "integrity, inspiring teaching, and devotion to medical students."

Young Margaret Thomson's interest in a medical career was evident early. In 1948, a reporter for the *Washington [PA] Daily News* highlighted the sixteen-year-old's summer work at the local hospital where she was gathering notes for a science paper: "If you'd peeped through windows of Garfield Hospital . . . you might have seen personable Margaret, who wants to study medicine . . . bent over a human body making notes for a pathologist. Her observations on the value of post-mortems were tucked in her paper, 'Life from Death.'"

In 1949, Margaret graduated Phi Beta Kappa with a bachelor's degree from Swarthmore College and immediately began her medical studies at the University of Rochester. With the awarding of her medical degree in 1953, she embarked on her pediatric internship at St. Louis City Hospital in Missouri. Post-graduate training in Houston, Texas, came next; a pediatric residency at Baylor University Affiliated Hospitals culminated in a chief residency in pediatrics at Jefferson Davis Hospital. In 1956, she completed a fellowship in pediatric cardiology at Baylor and Houston's Texas Children's Hospital.

Dr. Colgan returned to the UR School of Medicine and Dentistry in 1957 as an instructor in Pediatrics and director of pediatric education at St. Mary's Hospital. It was the beginning of a distinguished career that would extend over nearly four decades, inspiring generations of trainees, and providing care and comfort to thousands of children and their families.

All this was accomplished while Dr. Colgan was building a successful domestic life as wife of anesthesiologist Dr. Frank Colgan and mother of five children. It was a sign of the times that Meg and Frank, both UR medical students, were required to get the dean's permission before they could marry, a social rule that caused independent Meg some irritation.

That independence reappeared in 1971 when Meg, who was working 8 a.m. to 3:30 p.m., approached the department chair for additional compensation. In a personal letter to Meg, the dean conceded that "there may be some discrimination," but "we have made certain allowances because of your family commitments." His To-whom-it-may-concern letter in her personnel files agrees that her salary was "neither started nor advanced proportionately as high as other faculty of similar rank, who [work full-time] . . . Indeed, [her work] has been of very high quality and is extremely important, but family responsibilities plus the duties in the pediatric department are at times mutually exclusive." Dr. Colgan's daughter Ann Purcell notes that her father was much more annoyed by the results of the request than her mother.

In 1977, the Department of Pediatrics house staff were stressed by what they considered an "unnecessary diffusion of house staff and faculty" between the Genesee Hospital and RGH. The group sent a formal letter to Dr. Colgan, then pediatrician-in-chief at the Genesee Hospital, expressing their dissatisfaction with the situation, but praising her support as they expressed "our unending gratitude . . . for your excellent teaching and warm support. We need more teachers like you, Meg . . ."

When Dr. Elizabeth McAnarney presented Dr. Colgan with an Award of Merit from the Rochester Academy of Medicine in 1992, she noted that Dr. Colgan had been eagerly sought after as she moved from hospital to hospital—and that she was often the "doctor of choice" of UR faculty, house staff, and medical students when their own children needed medical care.

When asked recently how she met the challenges of raising five children, Dr. Colgan's response was simple: "It wasn't easy." Somehow, daughter Ann recalls, her mother always found time to fill the house with medical students and residents, eager for conversation and the home-cooked meals Meg loved to provide. A Cub Scout den mother and Girl Scout troop leader, Meg was also an avid cyclist, who enjoyed several European biking tours as well as cross-country skiing adventures. In retirement, she often volunteered at one of Rochester's city clinics. A voracious reader, she expanded her art history studies later in life and became a docent at UR's Memorial Art Gallery.

Dr. Colgan was a member of the American Academy of Pediatrics, the Rochester Academy of Medicine, and the Rochester Pediatric Society, as well as the honorary societies Phi Beta Kappa, Sigma Xi, and Alpha Omega Alpha. Dr. Colgan was first author of two articles in *Journal of Pediatrics*.

Her resume is certain proof that the career in science that young Meg Thomson sought found rich fulfillment. The fond remembrances of former students, colleagues, and friends are testimony to Meg's joyful spirit and to a life full of love of family, service, and dedication to her profession.

Note

1. The author extends thanks to Ann Purcell for providing background information on her mother's life.

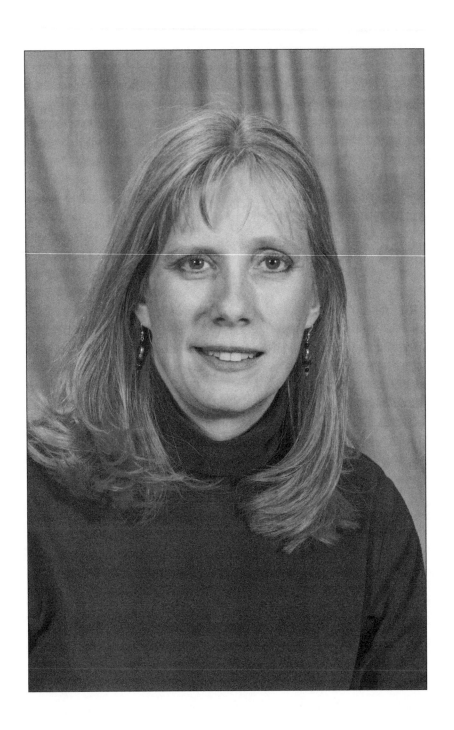

Chapter Ten

HEIDI V. CONNOLLY, MD

A traveler usually begins a journey with a firm endpoint in mind. Often, interesting signposts along the way may reshape the carefully planned itinerary. Yet, the fortunate traveler may find, at journey's end, both satisfaction and joy in achieving a destination that is totally unexpected.

"When I entered Northwestern University, I expected to be an electrical engineer, like my father, who loved his work," says Heidi Connolly, MD. "I had no idea what 'being a doctor' meant, although I respected the healthcare support given to my dad, whose career ended with complications from Type 1 diabetes."

Dr. Connolly's own career journey has not followed a straight line. But as she progressed from an undergraduate year in engineering at Northwestern University through specialty training in pediatric intensive care medicine, pediatric pulmonary medicine, and sleep medicine, she eventually reached a career destination that she says fits her perfectly. As director of the UR's Pediatric Sleep Medicine Program, her work is highly people-interactive, challenging, clinically interesting—and comprehensive in ways that enable her to combine clinical care with teaching for residents and post-graduate fellows.

"That's one of the best things about the UR Medical Center culture," she says, "and Pediatrics in particular. The leaders hire people who show promise of future success—and then they provide both freedom and support to help them grow into their career."

It was an alarming case of meningococcal meningitis contracted during her first year in the Honors Program for Medical Education at Northwestern that forced Connolly to change course for the first time. "The ten days I spent in the Intensive Care Unit and those following kept me from my math classes," she says. "A sympathetic woman professor enabled me to drop math, rather than fail. That was the end of engineering for me." Connolly completed undergraduate work in 1984 for a bachelor's degree in science from the honors program and went directly into Northwestern's medical school, from which she graduated in 1988.

As an undergraduate, Heidi had taken a highly unusual part-time job, one related in a curious way to her interest in obstetrics and gynecology. The Chicago Zoo had a female gorilla who staff veterinarians hoped would become pregnant. Over the years, the huge primate had been trained to urinate in a potty. Every day, before classes, Heidi would stop at the zoo and pick up a plastic cup of brown gorilla urine and deliver it to the laboratory, where signs of the hairy female's menstrual cycle would be analyzed. "This was my first lesson in reproductive endocrinology," says Heidi, with a laugh. (She was so attached to the gorilla and the zoo staff that she continued the job when she began medical school.)

Another potential course-changer appeared during Heidi's second year in medical school, when still another round of didactic classes found her fidgeting in her seat. She took her case to the dean, saying "This just isn't for me. I'm an action person. I like doing things, not listening." The dean pointed out that leaving without a medical degree would seriously compromise her future. She listened. A few months later when she began her clinical rotations, she was grateful for his tough talk. "I loved the rotations," she says. "I decided I would be a gynecologic oncologist."

The road sign to pediatrics appeared during Heidi's third-year rotation at Children's Memorial Hospital in Chicago. There she worked with two senior residents, young men who so clearly enjoyed their work and who were so effective in treating patients that they became role models. "Watching them working so joyfully and so independently really influenced my decision to choose pediatrics, even though that meant changing all my fourth-year electives," says Dr. Connolly.

Through her work in reproductive endocrinology, Connolly found two male mentors, Robert Chatterton, PhD, director of the reproductive endocrinology laboratory, and neonatologist Edward Ogata, MD. "Both Bob and Ed took me under their wings and talked with me about how to build a career that could be both meaningful and enjoyable," she recalls, noting that, because of them, she stayed on at Children's Hospital as a resident and then chief resident.

In 1992 Dr. Connolly began a three-year fellowship in critical care at the University of Chicago's Wyler Children's Hospital. For eight months during each of those years, she worked every other night on-call, in addition to her daytime hours. Support came from fellowship director Dr. Brian Rudinsky. "Brian understood the stresses that come with long hours working in the Intensive Care Unit (ICU), where the margin of error is zero. He made sure we all stayed grounded and emotionally secure," she says. In the laboratory, Connolly's research focused on blood flow distribution in critically ill patients, the mechanisms that tell the body where blood is needed, and how that decision is made.

There were few women physician-mentors during Heidi's post-graduate days. An exception was the director of the ICU at Children's Hospital. "Zehava Noah was the best clinician I have ever seen and the singular reason that I focused on ICU medicine at that time," she says. "Dr. Noah had so much clinical experience that she could see what was going to happen in the course of a patient's illness before anyone else recognized its possibility."

Were there gender issues that Heidi Connolly confronted during her early years in medicine? Her response to that question is simple: "I never looked for them. I never expected them. I never found them." Had the issues been there, Connolly would have dealt with them. As she did with the Ivy League interviewer who asked, "Why would a woman like you want a degree in science?" "I was so smokin' mad I wrote to the Admission's Office and demanded they refund my $20 application fee," she says. She got it.

Dr. Connolly arrived in Rochester to begin her fellowship in pediatric pulmonology in 1995. The invitation came from her former colleague at Children's

Hospital, Dr. Jeffrey Rubenstein; he had been an attending there when she was a resident. With the offer came a part-time job as an attending in Strong's ICU, where she used experience she had gained in Chicago. Three years later, Connolly was directing the pediatric critical care fellowship program.

"I love the intensity that comes with working in critical care. But I came to realize that I wanted to work with patients over the long term," Connolly explains. During a rotation in the adult sleep clinic, she met patients with sleep apnea and other medical problems producing breathing problems. Here was a group of people she could work with on a long-term basis. Included among the patients were a few children, whose numbers grew as the service expanded. In pediatric pulmonology, she had found her professional niche.

Now, as chief of the Division of Pediatric Sleep Medicine, Connolly directs the off-campus Pediatric Sleep Clinic, which last year saw 4,000 visits and completed 1,500 sleep studies. The clinic's white-painted walls are decorated with the colorful, signed handprints of children who have completed their study. Among them are several youngsters on the autism spectrum, whose medication-caused weight-gain has resulted in pulmonary issues, such as sleep apnea. Now Dr. Connolly is a principal collaborating investigator for the Autism Treatment Network, a multi-site collaborative trial on the effectiveness of iron treatment for insomnia in children with autism spectrum disorders.

At Golisano Children's Hospital, Dr. Connolly is a staff pulmonologist. Child psychiatry fellows rotating through the sleep clinic are mentored by Dr. Connolly. Within her profession, she is a member of the American Academy of Sleep Medicine, American Thoracic Society, a past member of the Society of Critical Care Medicine, and the Autism Intervention Research Network on Physical Health. She is also an elected member of Best Doctors in America.

Find a mentor. That's Dr. Connolly's advice for young people beginning their medical career. She has had several, including Dr. Susan Hyman, UR's chief of Developmental and Behavioral Pediatrics. "When I was in midcareer, Susan helped me determine my next move. She said, 'Let's make some research things happen here' and she did. Then, when I became a division chief, she talked with me about what it takes to be a leader."

Along with finding a mentor, make it a priority to find a life outside medicine. Heidi has been an active volunteer within her children's activities (Irish dancing and soccer). As a single mother, she has involved her children in the hard, but satisfying, work of restoring a Victorian home. "The work involves a lot of physical activity and results in a real product we can all enjoy," she says. (Restoration also involves engineering skills, which often remind Heidi of her father's profession and her early career goal.)

"Be open. And be a good citizen. Step up to the plate when you're needed," says Connolly. As for combining career and family, she cautions: "It's hard. There's no way around that. Find good friends, people you can talk to—and make it reciprocal. Help them when they need a hand." Dr. Connolly has three children: Margaret, a medicine/pediatric resident at URMC; William, who is working on a master's degree in finance at Boston College; and Andrew, a student at McQuaid High School. "Each of them is finding their own path, and each is succeeding in their own way," says their proud mother.

Finally, Dr. Connolly adds, to be successful in your career, you have to have the right motivation and the right people supporting you as you work to find your own path. Connolly's path has taken her far from what she imagined as a young medical student. The journey has been eventful, with unexpected turns along the way, and the destination is full of satisfactions.

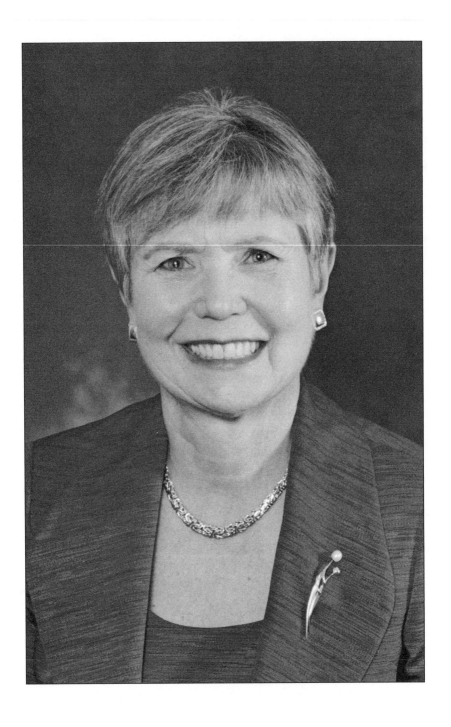

Chapter Eleven

Anne B. Francis, MD

"Follow your dream." That's the advice Dr. Anne Francis gives to young people, especially those looking to enter the medical profession. She's made it work for her, as signified by the gratitude of generations of Monroe County families and her thirteen-year listing as one of the "Best Doctors in America." At Rochester's venerable Elmwood Pediatric Group, Dr. Francis combined her skilled care for children with support for parents facing the difficult challenges that come with the "growing-up" years.

For twenty years, Dr. Francis was the Elmwood Group's managing partner, working to develop guidelines to help practicing pediatricians administer offices that are both efficient and financially viable. Currently she is focused on issues of quality care, serving as the URMC's representative for Solutions for Pediatric Safety, an initiative of several children's hospitals.

"Anne is compassionate, energetic, and brilliant," says Elmwood Group partner Dr. Carolyn Cleary. "She's always up to date on advances in medicine, bringing the best care to patients. A strong advocate for children *and* pediatricians, she's been a wonderful mentor to me."

A woman dedicated to expanding horizons, Dr. Francis also has made teaching, research, leadership within her profession, and community service important and life-enriching components of her career.

Dr. Francis says she came of age at the right time. Growing up during the sixties in a small city in western Pennsylvania, she was part of a generation for whom the future seemed open, the rigidities of the fifties exploded by new social norms. "We thought this was a new world," she says, "one where we could do anything we wanted to do."

But was it *really* that easy? Of course, not. As a young woman who had shined during her undergraduate years (a fine student and president of her sorority), she encountered real-life social challenges during her four years in medical school at the University of Pittsburgh. They involved demographics, specifically gender and racial issues. "In a class of 110, four of us were women, ten of the men were black," she recalls, disproportions that she couldn't ignore. "As a woman, I was often made to feel that I didn't belong there," she recalls. "More than one [male student] said, 'You took a place that should have been given to my friend.' Another: 'I should date you. You have good earning potential.'" Change was on the way, however. After Dr. Francis's freshman year in medical school, the number of women in the incoming class increased from four to twenty-five.

As for gender bias, "The women who preceded me had a much more dramatic experience [with discrimination] than I did," says Dr. Francis. Still, bias was a shadowy presence during Dr. Francis's residency and internship years at the University of North Carolina at Chapel Hill. At that time, UNC used a pyramid system to "weed out" medical trainees not meeting the highest standards. At Saturday rounds soon after Francis's arrival, the department chair bluntly announced, "Some of you will be asked to leave." Francis learned that the previous year two women in the group of eight residents had been dropped from the program. Was it *because* they were women? she wondered. "I was so worried I went immediately to the chairman—who quickly reassured me." With this experience, a helpful lesson was learned: Being forthright and outspoken about your concerns is often key to eliminating a troubling situation.

Many other challenges would be met and overcome during Dr. Francis's long career. But it was during these early years that she honed the skills that have led to both professional success and a satisfying life in medicine: hard work, determination, a gift for analysis, a cooperative spirit, and—not least—a cheerful outlook and a hearty laugh.

As a teenager in Elwood City, Anne had discovered her passion for medicine through the sixties' equivalent of social media: weekly encounters with friends in front of the TV set with "Young Dr. Kildare." A pre-med summer research internship in pathology made possible by the pharmaceutical company Smith, Kline & French cemented her interest when she was assigned to do her research in Children's Hospital in Pittsburgh. "Although dissecting kidneys was not one of my successes," she says, "the exposure to this amazing hospital and its staff showed me that pediatrics would be my career path."

After four years as a chemistry major at Thiel College in Greenville, Pennsylvania, Anne began her medical training at the University of Pittsburgh School of Medicine and its independent children's hospital. There she found a mentor in the chair of pediatrics, Dr. Thomas Kevin Oliver. "Tim was a Pied Piper who showed me my first clinical case, a child with chicken pox." Another mentor, Dr. Robert Hingson, had developed the epidural block. Hingson, then head of obstetrics anesthesiology at Magee Women's Hospital in Pittsburgh, had also invented the jet injector, and Anne became a member of a team that went into the Pittsburgh community to immunize children against rubella.

As an active member of the Student Medical Association at Pittsburgh, Anne met Charlie Francis, who was preparing for a career in hematology. (She was impressed when he volunteered to write a committee report, a job she—the only woman on the committee—had expected to inherit.) Anne and Charlie married at the end of their junior year and later couples-matched to UNC/Chapel Hill, she in pediatrics, he in internal medicine.

As the final year of their residencies approached, Anne and Charlie looked to the immediate future. The University of Rochester loomed large. Charlie was interested in coagulation and the UR has one of the best fellowships in that field. Dr. Floyd Denny, UNC's chair of pediatrics and an expert in streptococcal infections, introduced Anne to UR's Dr. Caren Hall, also an infectious disease specialist. So was Hall's father, the distinguished Rochester pediatrician Dr. Burtis Breese of the Elmwood Pediatric Group. Here was a perfect segue into clinical practice for Anne.

"Charlie and I arrived in Rochester in 1976, to start our careers, buy our first house, and pregnant with our first child," she says. She soon joined the

Elmwood Pediatric Group, working part-time. The group had deep ties within the Rochester community; in addition to Dr. Breese, its partners included Drs. Frank Disney, William Talpey, John Green, and later Dr. Michael Pichichero, who brought to the practice a strong interest in research.

During those years, Elmwood Pediatrics was providing care for infants born at Highland Hospital. There Anne Francis met Dr. Ruth Lawrence, medical director of the nursery, who became her first female mentor. ("Get a long cord for your telephone," Dr. Lawrence advised.)

"I soon realized I could be a real asset to the group," she says. "At that time, many women were entering professions and having families. There were few role models for them. Many of these new professional women were facing the challenges of having their first child without the benefit of family nearby and not all had good support systems. They needed someone to guide them through this transition. I had walked that walk and I knew what their stresses were." Dr. Francis made time to talk with these mothers, encouraging them to look for extra help in the home when it was needed, as she had. "One of the cornerstones of my philosophy is this: if our children are going to receive good care at home, we have to support those who are taking care of them."

Early in her career, Dr. Francis had been appalled by the number of children brought to the office with head injuries after bicycle accidents. Protective helmets were rarely used by cyclists in those days, and bike accidents were frequent and often disastrous. Partnering with Pittsford pediatrician Dr. Gregory Eldredge, Dr. Francis initiated and promoted a bike-helmet safety campaign which grew into a comprehensive citywide bicycle-safety coalition of pediatricians, bicycle shop owners, Blue Cross Blue Shield, and parents. The effort soon went statewide, with Dr. Francis at the helm of the American Academy of Pediatrics (AAP) campaign in the entire upstate area.

Research was becoming an important part of the Elmwood Group's work during the early 1980s and '90s. "This was what I had hoped for," says Dr. Francis, "a clinical practice with a strong research effort. I learned so much during those years: how to enroll patients, what studies work in a clinical situation and what didn't." Drs. Breese and Disney had done much of the original practice-based research on streptococcal disease. Later, based on that experience, the group was poised to help with many new vaccine trials, including the revolutionary vaccine for *Hemophilus influenzae b* (Hib), a disease that was killing or disabling thousands of children every year. (When brought to market, the vaccine eventually reduced childhood death rate from Hib by 90 percent.) Other vaccine trials in which the group participated were those for acellular diphtheria, pertussis, tetanus vaccine (DPT), rotavirus, nasal flu, and several combination vaccines.

Dr. Francis continued to work on vaccine trials, including studies of streptococcal disease and otitis media, as well as issues related to healthcare costs. As the numbers and cost of vaccines increased, she saw their impact on the office budget, and she worked to develop recognition of that fact within the profession. Her name now appears on forty scientific papers and publications, often as first author.

Throughout these years Dr. Francis worked, worked, and then worked more. In addition to taking care of her Elmwood Group patients, she became a preceptor for UR medical students and residents, and for some years she supervised the nursery at Highland Hospital. Often, she was called out of bed in the middle of the night, and she worked most weekends. What made it all possible was the Elmwood Group's flexible scheduling policy, which allowed her time to be involved in her children's schooling and activities.

In 1978 she became a full partner in the Elmwood Pediatric Group.

In the late 1980s, Dr. Francis attended her first AAP Women's Leadership Conference for board-certified women pediatricians in San Francisco. "It was an eye-opening moment," she says. "I met many of the 'super women' in my field, women who were making a mark nationally in healthcare." That trip sparked her interest in what she calls "organizational pediatrics" That interest has been deep and abiding, as attested by a resume that lists her name as chair, vice president, or member of seventeen AAP-related organizations.

During these years she has supported methods to improve practice management and efforts to help pediatricians meet challenging changes in payment methods.

For fourteen years Dr. Francis has been a member of the UR Medical Center Board and currently serves on its Advancement Committee and Joint Committee on Quality of Care. Chief among her many other professional affiliations are those related to the AAP: president, NY Chapter 1, District 11; and treasurer, NY District II; chair, Project Advisory Committee, Childhood Immunization Support Program; chair, Private Payer Advocacy Advisory Committee; and chair, Editorial Committee, Practice Management Online. She has also been deeply involved with the work of the Rochester Academy of Medicine and with the Monroe County Medical Society, and she is currently medical director of the Mary Cariola Children's Center.

In 2007, Dr. Francis received both the Edward Mott Moore Award from the Monroe County Medical Society and the Charles Vanchiere Award from the AAP.

There is, for most doctors, a life beyond—yet enhanced by—their profession as physicians. Dr. Anne Francis is strongly rooted in the greater Rochester community, in part as an elder and trustee of the Pittsford Presbyterian Church. She says her greatest pride is not in her own achievements, but in those of her adult offspring: David, a surgeon at Vanderbilt University; Katherine, a former Marshall Fellow at Oxford, now helping develop strategic plans for not-for-profit organizations; and Peter, an investment banker in the medical sector in San Francisco.

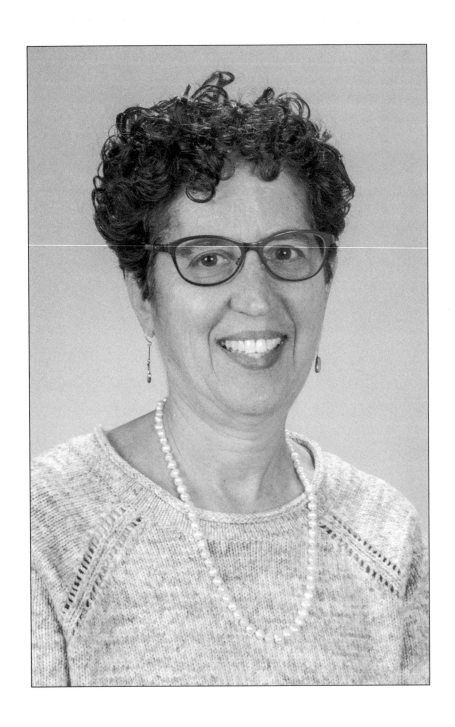

Chapter Twelve

Lynn C. Garfunkel, MD

Dr. Lynn Garfunkel believes she's the luckiest physician in the whole Department of Pediatrics, and that's a very big department. Certainly, if variety is the spice of life, Lynn's professional schedule provides plenty of it—not just at one medical center, but two.

More than eighty young doctors advancing through their residency training in pediatrics or internal medicine-pediatrics are guided, in part, each year by this lively and friendly preceptor. Thanks to the healthcare partnership between the University of Rochester School of Medicine and Dentistry (URSMD), Rochester General Hospital, and Rochester Regional Health (RRH), Dr. Garfunkel is often on the road traveling between two hospitals, two sets of conference rooms, and two clinics.

"I work with two amazing groups, colleagues and residents. I may be a teacher, but I learn so much from the residents," she says. "And I still have the privilege of seeing patients. Every day for me is different. One of the great pleasures of this job is seeing your learners become empathic practitioners and thoughtful educators."

Not all of Dr. Garfunkel's career has been spent in academia. Community outreach has been a big part of her life. She has been an advisor for Rochester's Baden Street Settlement House; a volunteer physician for Mercy Outreach Center (formerly Corpus Christi); and secretary for Families Advocating Music Education. She traveled to earthquake-torn Haiti in 2010 and again in 2015, where she worked as a volunteer physician and medical educator.

Lynn's father was an academic, a professor of physics at the University of Pittsburgh. If he represented science, her mother, a weaver and ceramicist, brought the arts into focus for Lynn. When Lynn was in sixth grade, the family spent a sabbatical year at the University of Cambridge, where they lived in the spacious wing of a house built as a wedding present for Charles Darwin's granddaughter. The owners, an immunologist and a geriatrician, lent their own scientific stamp to Lynn's early years; the experience was reinforced when, as a teenager, Lynn twice returned to Cambridge alone to spend summers working as a nanny for these British friends.

Tufts University in Massachusetts was the undergraduate college of choice for Lynn, who chose to major in child development and biology. Garfunkel quickly became deeply intellectually involved in Tufts's excellent child development program; she was particularly attracted to learning how the young brain matures. But as her senior year approached, the future still seemed uncertain: would she be a special education teacher, a psychologist, or something else? A doctor back in Pittsburgh urged her to apply to medical school. His counsel found its mark, and Lynn took her MCAT exam at the beginning of her senior year, almost a year later than her classmates. In 1977, Dr. Lynn Garfunkel graduated from Tufts College, *magna cum laude*.

Lynn entered the Medical College of Pennsylvania in 1977, where she spent the next four years. In 1981, she began her pediatric internship and residency at Children's Hospital Medical Center in Cincinnati, and served as chief resident there from 1984 to 1985. For the next two years she worked as a primary care pediatrician in Cincinnati, before moving to Washington, DC.

Dr. Garfunkel spent the following three years at Children's National Medical Center as a clinical assistant professor of pediatrics, a faculty member of George Washington University. During this time she was awarded an NIH training grant in Medical Faculty Development at Michigan State University.

Dr. Garfunkel's relationship with the University of Rochester began in 1990, when, as a senior instructor, she began a two-year fellowship to continue her studies in general academic pediatrics. "I really came here as a faculty spouse," she says, with a big smile. In Cincinnati during training, she met Dr. Craig Orlowski, soon to be her husband, and followed him to Washington. In the late 1980s, department chair Dr. Robert Hoekelman and head of the search committee Dr. Elizabeth McAnarney were looking to expand the Pediatric Endocrinology Division. In hiring Dr. Orlowski, they met and also recruited his wife, Dr. Lynn Garfunkel. "I interviewed with our young son, Zach, on my back," Lynn recalls.

After making a second trip to Rochester to meet the faculty at RGH where general pediatrics was expanding, Lynn and Craig chose to move to Rochester. As a new young faculty member, she was assigned to work in the hospital's inpatient unit, the outpatient clinics, and in the newborn nursery; as a fellow, she continued pursuing her graduate courses at the UR. In her early years as a fellow, she also spent time in the pediatric clinic at Strong Memorial Hospital. Her association with both hospitals continues. As a primary care pediatrician and preceptor at Rochester General Pediatric Associates, she also spends time in the newborn nursery at RGH.

A major part of Dr. Garfunkel's positions as clinician-educator is training and mentoring residents and fellows in both pediatrics at Golisano Children's Hospital (GCH), RGH, and in the combined internal medicine-pediatrics practice at Culver Medical Group. As preceptor, she listens and observes as residents present relevant information about and to their patients. But she does not just observe the facts; she is alert to the ever-present and implicit "silent curriculum": What is the presenter's attitude? How is she or he relating to the patient? Is she or he a good model of pediatric professionalism? What are his or her analytic skills?

Each year, Dr. Garfunkel helps recruit sixteen new pediatric and eight new internal medicine-pediatric residents from more than 250 invited applicants. Mentoring and advising are both important, as Garfunkel knows. She credits her early violin teachers for showing her that dedication to craft can bring satisfaction to both teacher and learner. She's learned much from her own program director and early pediatric educators, but also much from her first pediatric chairs in Rochester, Dr. Robert Hoekelman and Dr. Elizabeth McAnarney.

Dr. Garfunkel herself has mentored many young people coming into the profession. Dr. Sarah Collins-McGowan, lead physician at Genesee Pediatrics, is one of those mentees. She says, "over the past ten years, Lynn has been an incredibly important mentor in both my professional career and my personal development. Her mentorship style is much like parenting—she steadfastly believes in my abilities, but will be honest if I'm on the wrong track. That kind of grounding is critical to the young physician who is building her confidence and skills. Having her acknowledge a job well done is a great feeling."

"I've enjoyed teaching from the time I was 'big sister' to my siblings at home," Lynn says. In fact, the honor she values most is the Academic Mentoring Award she received at URMC in 2014. One special interest now is her work on the twelve-member Pediatric Residency Review Committee of the Accreditation Council of Graduate Medical Education, which not only accredits pediatric training programs, but strives to improve and disseminate innovative teaching methods appropriate to a new generation of learners.

As a pediatric educator and primary care clinician serving a predominantly underserved community, Dr. Garfunkel's scope extends well beyond the UR to the national and international community of academic educators. She served on the steering committee for Global Health Educators, as well as the board of the Association of Pediatric Program Directors (APPD). A fellow of the American Academy of Pediatrics, Garfunkel has also been active in the Academic Pediatric Association (APA), as a regional research chair for CORNET, the Continuity Research Network; a facilitator in the Educational Scholar Program; and for more than twelve years on the steering committee for the continuity clinic special interest group of the APA. She is deeply involved with the APPD, whose mission is "leading the advancement of education to ensure the health and well-being of children."

As an invited lecturer, her most recent presentations have been at the Pediatric Academic Society's annual meeting in Baltimore, the AAP meeting on Mental Health, and in 2017 at the APPD annual meeting preconference seminar, all involving how best to train pediatric residents and psychology postdoctoral fellows in caring for children and families with behavioral and mental health needs in primary care.

Lynn and Craig have "two amazing kids": daughter Rachel works in Chicago for the Toronto-based social action organization, "WE," and Zachary is a global product manager for a medical supply company in Seattle. High praise from Lynn goes to husband Craig, who has always shared in 50 percent of all home and family endeavors. She says, "It's been a great ride!"

Balancing work and career can be tricky. "It's a juggling act. Sometimes a ball gets dropped—and sometimes something breaks. It helps to have among your family, friends, and colleagues people who can help you move through hairy situations. I'm so fortunate in that, really, almost everything has worked out," she says. "I thoroughly enjoy what I do—working with my patients, my residents, my colleagues—and I am so proud of all their achievements and successes. I've earned people's trust. And I've learned that self-determination is really important."

Dr. Garfunkel's advice for young people coming into the profession is based on lessons learned in her own career:

- There are many paths within our profession. Find paths that will best suit your temperament and talents. When opportunities arise, be thoughtful and consider your options.
- Have fun and embrace challenges.
- Strive to develop competency, relationships, and autonomy.
- Get involved with pediatrics at the national level. You'll find friends and colleagues who will enrich your perspective and offer good counsel away from the office.
- Remember: you can't cure everyone, but you can certainly *help* many.
- Above all, enjoy!

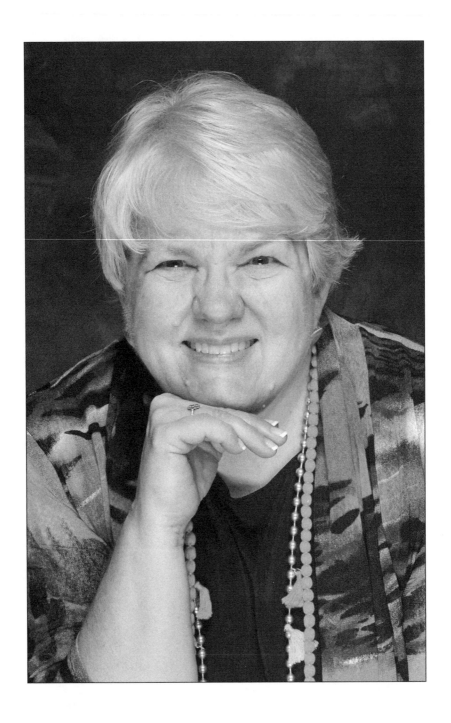

Chapter Thirteen

CATHERINE A. GOODFELLOW, MD

The upward career path forged by Catherine A. Goodfellow, MD, could stand as a non-traditional model for anyone considering the many possibilities of a life in medicine. Goodfellow was a licensed nurse, married three years to her high school sweetheart, and had a view to the future when she entered medical school at the University of Buffalo in 1979.

Today, the firm she founded, Genesis Pediatrics, includes eight pediatricians, three nurse practitioners, and a total staff of nearly fifty. In its offices on Elmgrove Road in the town of Gates, New York, west of Rochester, Genesis recorded over 28,000 patient visits in 2016.

"I did my research," Dr. Goodfellow says of Genesis's beginnings. "I visited OB/GYN offices throughout the area west of Rochester and looked at the availability of pediatric services. After assessing the situation, it was clear that we could serve a need, that parents were looking for quality care for their children in a convenient west side location." With advice and support from her husband, Alan, a Kodak engineer, Cathy Goodfellow drew up a business plan. She began small—herself and a medical secretary working in half-a-house in Gates. The new pediatric office—Genesis Pediatrics, LLC, symbol of birth and beginnings, was incorporated on July 5, 1988.

Cathy grew up in Hollidaysburg, a small town in the mountains of central Pennsylvania, where her father was a family doctor. A Korean War veteran, he had entered Grove City College using the GI Bill in September 1954, ten days before Cathy was born. Three years later, he and his family moved to Philadelphia, where he began his medical studies at Temple University.

With his medical degree realized, Cathy's father moved the family back to Hollidaysburg, where he became both an attending physician at nearby Altoona Hospital and a charter member of the American Academy of Family Practitioners.

It was the 1950s and Cathy's mother had her own expectations: "My mother said she would care for him and the children, cook, and 'keep house,' but she wouldn't work outside the house to support him," Cathy recalls. Consequently, her father, who was also a licensed funeral director, worked nights in the local funeral home to supplement their income. (Cathy remembers playing tag in the basement among the caskets when she was young.)

Throughout high school in Hollidaysburg, Cathy envisioned going to medical school; she loved making house calls with her father. "I wanted to become a doctor, but I fell in love with my husband, who I'd known since the second grade," she says. Medical school at that time seemed a far reach. Instead she chose nursing, and enrolled in Altoona Hospital's School of Nursing. Cathy says she loved the clinical work in the hospital, but when a baccalaureate nursing program opened at Pennsylvania State University in Hershey with a link to Altoona, she eagerly signed on.

Three years later, Cathy received her nursing degree, and soon after she married Alan, who had just graduated from Carnegie Mellon University in Pittsburgh. With an offer from Kodak for the young electrical engineer, the couple headed north towards Rochester, now and then looking wistfully out the car's back window toward their disappearing mountain home.

Once settled in their apartment in Rochester, Cathy looked for a place to use her new nursing skills. She found an ideal situation in the Newborn Nursery at Highland Hospital. There she met Dr. Ruth Lawrence, director of the nursery, who was becoming well known as a lactation specialist.

Soon the young nurse was looking to expand her career options. "When I asked Dr. Lawrence about my going to medical school, she said, 'If you're serious, you'll have to leave nursing.'" Dr. Lawrence offered a new possibility: There was a research assistant position open in the Department of Pediatrics, a post that provided support for both Dr. Lawrence and Dr. Elizabeth McAnarney. (Dr. McAnarney at that time was deeply involved in the Rochester Adolescent Maternity Program [RAMP], designed to support urban teenage mothers and their babies with care and counseling.)

Both doctors were working on projects in their respective specialties: Dr. Lawrence's pioneering book on breastfeeding and Dr. McAnarney's research on adolescent mothers. "In addition to a lot of proofreading and reference-checking, I did much of the videotaping of the young women in the RAMP project and their babies," says Dr. Goodfellow.

During these three years, first at Highland Hospital and then within the Department of Pediatrics, Cathy Goodfellow made connections that would be important for her future. "I met most of the pediatricians in the area and many of the OB/GYN doctors," she says. After long discussions with her husband about the pros and cons of starting medical school, the die was cast. She would go for it—even though she would first have to take the necessary premed courses in physics, biochemistry, and statistics. A year later, she finished her course work: all As.

A huge disappointment followed—Cathy's first application to a medical school was rejected in spite of her solid academic record. She was devastated and angry. "I'll never forget the interviewer who told me, 'As a nurse, you're already in the medical profession.'" As if to say, stay where you are and be satisfied. (At that time, Dr. Goodfellow says, that medical school, like many others, accepted more students than they could handle and expected 20 percent of the underachievers to drop out.)

The next year, Cathy was accepted at the University of Buffalo School of Medicine, where she flourished, graduating in 1983. She had expected to specialize in family medicine, but in her third rotation chose pediatrics, in part because her conversations with Dr. Ruth Lawrence had emphasized the many satisfactions to be found working with children and their parents. "I had a wonderful experience at Buffalo, a school that accepted just enough students—and expected them all to graduate. I never would have been happy in a super-competitive atmosphere. We serve a big God, and He knows what we need."

With her goal of becoming a physician achieved, Dr. Goodfellow was thrilled in 1983 to be "matched" with Strong Memorial Hospital for her residency. With two sons now, and two more children to come, she took four years to complete her residency. (To ensure *some* control over her days, she volunteered to do the on-call scheduling for her class of residents, a task she continues at Genesis.)

In 1984, Dr. Goodfellow joined the small practice of a pediatrician in the neighboring community of Brighton, working one afternoon a week in his continuity of care clinic and one afternoon at a Strong Memorial clinic. Later, with expansion plans in hand, the Brighton doctor doubled his staff, hiring two additional pediatricians to join the practice, but space was limited and by 1988 a change was needed.

Cathy began researching possibilities for an independent practice on the west side of Rochester in the growing community of Gates, near the family's home. Once convinced of the need, she and her husband charted the plan to develop Genesis Pediatrics, deliberately choosing a name that was not linked to a particular person or location. Its logo: an apple.

Genesis soon outgrew its beginnings in that half-a-house on Buffalo Road. Three months later, they moved into a newly completed professional building which would be the practice's home for a decade, from 1989 to 1999. And still the practice grew. Genesis Pediatrics pediatricians and nurse practitioners have moved twice more, and now see patients at their new suite of offices on Elmgrove Road.

Genesis Pediatrics is now nearly thirty years old, and, like the Goodfellow children, it has grown into something far more than was ever expected. Cathy has some pride, but much more thankfulness, for the life that pediatrics has provided her and her family.

She has some cautionary advice for those looking to enter the field. First, if you have a life partner, be sure you both are in agreement about the wisdom of choosing medicine and have some understanding of its demands. "Pediatrics is not a nine-to-five job. Sickness doesn't take holidays—and you'll be working on some of them," she points out. Parents of sick children can be demanding; they're worried and want you to "fix it," a goal that may be difficult to achieve.

Dr. Goodfellow understands the time stresses faced by mothers in medicine who have children. Two of her children were born while she was in medical school, two more during her residency, and there was no family living nearby to help. She's experienced those stresses.

"If you want to do clinical pediatrics only for the paycheck, you may be choosing the wrong thing," she warns. She points out the recent reductions in reimbursements, changing payment methodologies for procedures and services, and escalating mandatory reporting and record keeping. ("Remember, I have to support the fifty people who work for me," she says.) As CEO of Genesis, Goodfellow herself continues to see patients four days a week.

Dr. Goodfellow sees the role of the independent physician slowly disappearing. "More than 50 percent of this year's residents will be employed by others," she says. With that, she fears some loss of commitment to practice. "We care more about the things that we're personally invested in, and we tend not to put ourselves out for someone else's business," she says. "Putting yourself out," giving more than is required, is a quality that doctors traditionally have been known for. Dr. Goodfellow wonders: can young members of the profession, with different expectations, be comfortable with that?

As for herself, she is deeply grateful for her success. "I never would have thought I'd be running such a large practice when we started out, that our little practice would thrive—in pediatrics, of all things," she says. Now, thirty years after its small beginnings, Genesis has brought its founder enormous satisfaction. "It's gratifying to see patients whose mothers were former patients," she says with pride.

As it turned out, Cathy Goodfellow has been involved in family medicine, her first love, all these many years. And her own children—Jordan in Denver; David and Andrea in the Rochester area; and Aaron in Anchorage, Alaska—have a mother of whose entrepreneurial accomplishments they can be proud.

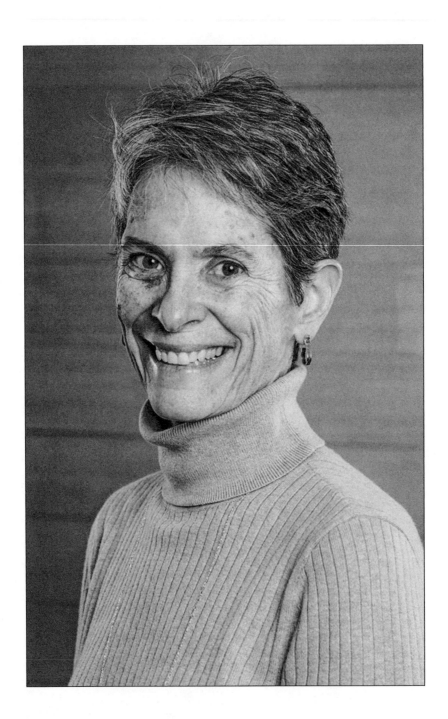

Chapter Fourteen

Ronnie Guillet, MD, PhD

Dr. Ronnie Guillet's career is marked by honors. Yet her advice to young people hoping to become doctors is surprisingly simple: "Show up—and pay attention." Five simple words, important for everyone. But they're delivered with backup: "Always have your antennae waving, looking for possibilities."

Young Dr. Ronnie Guillet certainly was alert on the day in 1983 when she was interviewing for a fellowship in neonatology at the Children's Hospital of Pennsylvania, waiting for an elevator at the hospital of the University of Pennsylvania. She struck up a conversation with a woman also waiting at the elevator door. The woman happened to be Dr. Maria Delavoria-Papadopoulos, one of the "grandmothers of neonatology," who had famously saved some premature babies with breathing problems by using a primitive ventilator in the days before surfactant therapy.

"I was in Philadelphia then because my husband Ernest, then an ophthalmology resident, was interviewing for a fellowship at the Wills Eye Institute. We were looking for a city where we both could pursue our subspecialty training," Dr. Guillet recalls. By the end of that spontaneous conversation with Dr. Papadopoulos, the job problem had resolved. "I'd love to have you come to work as a fellow in my lab," the eminent doctor said to the young researcher.

"That was total serendipity," Guillet insists, the kind of twist of fate that she values. While some young people identify their career goals early and move ahead single-mindedly, Dr. Guillet sees value in remaining flexible, ready to respond to unexpected circumstances which may have great potential . . . like that moment when she met an important mentor at the door of an elevator in a strange city.

Ronnie Guillet arrived in Rochester in 1973 after graduating from State University of New York (SUNY) Albany with a degree in Biology. "I never intended to be a doctor," she says. Her plan was to be a research scientist, and her goal was to pursue a PhD in the Department of Radiation Biology and Biophysics, working with UR's Saul Michaelson, DVM, on the hazards of microwaves. Michaelson specifically was looking for endocrine markers in rats. Here, in his lab, Guillet's interest in the development of the central nervous system was fostered, a curiosity that would eventually transfer from animals to humans.

She also recalls the day in 1975 when, almost by chance, a fellow graduate student said, "Why don't you consider going to medical school? They're looking for women these days for the MD/PhD program." At that time, she was attending pediatric endocrinology clinics once a week with Dr. Gilbert Forbes, a pediatric endocrinologist and world-renowned expert in body composition and nutrition, who was a member of her thesis faculty. "You ask good questions," Dr. Forbes told her. "Why don't you apply?" Encouraged, she also met with Dr. Paul LaCelle, then chair of the Department of Radiation Biology and Biophysics. "After frankly sharing my career doubts, I had to convince both senior scientists—two weeks before the program deadline!—that I should be part of the program," Guillet recalls. She convinced them.

Uncertainty surfaced again during her first year in medical school. "I remember thinking, this is a big mistake," Guillet says, with a smile. "As a self-motivator, I didn't like to sit in a classroom and be taught." However, once the courses required more "thinking" than "memorization" medical school got better each year. In 1980, Dr. Guillet was awarded her MD/PhD degree from the University of Rochester, a labor-intensive project she completed in seven years.

Our life paths are rarely free from obstacles. Ronnie Guillet faced a major disappointment waiting for her pediatric residency match. She and Ernest were married, and that meant moving to San Francisco where Ernest would continue his training as an ophthalmology resident. The bad news was that Ronnie didn't match with the medical centers to which she'd applied. As a result, she says, "I felt like I was a reject wearing a scarlet letter" when she was accepted for a residency in pediatrics at Mt. Zion Hospital and Medical Center, now part of the University of California, San Francisco.

Chance, however, had turned up a favorable card, one of several that Guillet credits with helping advance her career. A conversation with UR physician/scientist Caren Hall led to a link with another of the "grandmothers of neonatology": Dr. Roberta Ballard, then chair of pediatrics and director of newborn services at Mt. Zion. Ballard has done groundbreaking research in preventing and treating chronic lung disease in premature infants. San Francisco was thus the ideal situation, Guillet says, an environment where she could experience the best of both worlds: bread-and-butter pediatrics and encouragement from one of the best neonatologists in the country.

She subsequently transferred to the University of California, San Francisco, for her third year of residency. "After an excellent grounding caring for 'horses,' I found myself in a place where I could learn from the 'zebras,'" she says.

A two-year fellowship in neonatal-perinatal medicine in the Children's Hospital of Philadelphia program led Dr. Guillet to the University of Pennsylvania School of Medicine in Philadelphia, where she worked with her "elevator-door mentor," Dr. Papadopoulos. At its completion, she faced another move, this time to Rochester. The good news at this point was that her husband had accepted a partnership there with an ophthalmological practice. For Ronnie, though, there was no open position in pediatrics. There *was* an intriguing opportunity, however, in the laboratory of Carol Kellogg, PhD, a basic scientist who was studying the effects of drugs on the brains of the offspring of drug-dosed pregnant rats. It paid to be flexible, Guillet discovered; after two-and-a-half years working in Dr. Kellogg's lab, she was awarded a major three-year NIH grant to pursue research on the possible effects of caffeine on neonatal rat brain development.

When the NIH grant ended in 1991, the question became: What next? Once again, a conversation provided the answer. Guillet made an appointment to talk with Dr. Dale Phelps, then chief of the UR Division of Neonatology. The answer to her question was quick in coming: Dr. Phelps suggested that she join the faculty as an assistant professor of pediatrics. She would be able to resume taking care of the critically ill infants in the Neonatal Intensive Care Unit, while still pursuing her basic science research involving brain development and injury in neonatal rats.

In 2007, Dr. Guillet was appointed professor of pediatrics at Strong Memorial Hospital (Neonatology), Highland Hospital, and Rochester General Hospital. Over the years, she has filled many roles at the URMC, including teaching and mentoring medical students, neonatal nurses, residents, and fellows. She has directed the Neonatal-Perinatal Fellowship Program and until recently was chief of the Department of Pediatrics at Highland Hospital. She has been an active reviewer for several professional journals, and her committee responsibilities have been extensive, both within the University of Rochester Medical Center and beyond, including chairing the Data Safety Monitoring Committee for two National Institutes of Neurological Disorders and Stroke (NINDS)-funded multicenter trials.

Dr. Guillet believes her greatest career accomplishment may be her ability to mentor young scientists and clinicians. There's strong evidence to support that: In 2010 she was awarded the Faculty Mentoring Award, a university-wide honor. Guillet says she enjoys "connecting people"—and she is always aware of how she has been helped by others.

Guillet sees the mentor-mentee relationship as an important two-way path; in guiding her mentees she has enriched her own career scope. One neonatology fellow with a specific interest in bilirubin was looking for a mentor. "I agreed to work with him and learned a lot in the process," she says. Another was focused on kidney injury; working with him, Guillet connected with an international group studying similar issues. As a result, she is a member of the Steering Committee of the Neonatal Kidney Collaborative and co-author of many publications from that group.

One of her mentees, Dr. Rita Dadiz, now associate director of the Neonatal-Perinatal Medicine Fellowship Program, says "Ronnie has been very important in my career development—now she's the role model for my own mentoring. She has that special quality of being very present when you're together, and an open-door policy that makes those meetings possible. You sense that she's committed to you, and that's a phenomenal strength."

"I've had fabulous women mentors," says Dr. Guillet, many more than could be covered in this interview. She took qualities from each that seemed right for her own life. Some of her mentors chose to give their lives to their careers, she says. "I didn't want that. I wanted more control over my own life." The result: a rich blend of career, marriage, family, and community involvement. Dr. Guillet says her proudest achievements are her two daughters, Alyson and Rebecca, one a resident in obstetrics and gynecology and one a lawyer. "Both are amazing, accomplished young women," she says with pride.

This woman, whose original goal was to become a research scientist, over the years has expanded her vision. Now, Dr. Ronnie Guillet believes that her greatest accomplishment may be this: she has become a life guide for dozens of young people who have turned to her, hoping to build successful lives in the challenging, many-faceted realm of medicine and science.

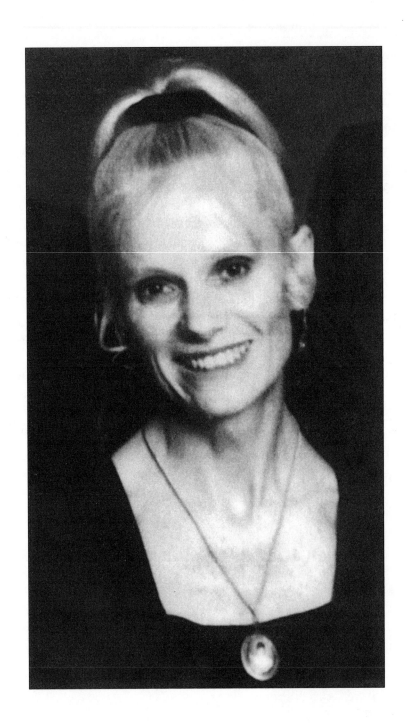

Chapter Fifteen

CAROLINE B. HALL, MD (1939–2012)[1]

In the annals of Rochester medicine few names shine brighter than that of Caroline (Caren) Breese Hall, internationally known for her groundbreaking work on the respiratory viruses that once claimed hundreds of thousands of young children.

Dr. Hall's seminal studies—more than five hundred—of Respiratory Syncytial Virus (RSV) and Human Herpesvirus-6 (HHV-6) changed the way pediatricians around the western world treat children with infectious diseases. Her early studies defined the diagnosis, epidemiology, transmission, and therapy of RSV bronchiolitis in children.

With her discovery that bronchiolitis, the clinical disease caused by RSV, spreads through hand and fomites contact, Caren's career took off like a rocket. Her name would soon become synonymous with RSV, whether in infants, children, young adults, the elderly, or high-risk groups. When HHV-6 was identified as the cause of Roseola, Dr. Hall became one of the first physicians in the country to track the clinical spectrum of the ubiquitous infection that causes one-third of complex febrile seizures and post-transplant encephalitis. Her later work focused on the possible relationship between genetics and the vertical transmission of the virus from mother to infant.

Dr. Hall early recognized that the clinician's office could be a perfect research laboratory, and she worked to build partnerships between pediatrics faculty and community pediatricians. Her outreach helped create the infrastructure of what is now known as the New Vaccine Surveillance Network, where community doctors work with University faculty to gauge the prevalence of community-wide diseases and chart the efficacy of the vaccines used to combat them.

"Caren had a sharp eye for discerning what sort of research was clinically significant and would have real pay-off in terms of advancing kids' health," said John Treanor, MD, recalling his early years as her student at URMC. Another trainee put it more succinctly, "I always figured she just never slept."

Within the medical school, Dr. Hall was revered as a clinician whose observational skills led her to the right diagnosis more often than not. As a teacher, she was known for her gift for reaching out to learners at every level; she won the pediatric house staff teaching award more than ten times.

Dr. Hall's life beyond the laboratory was rich. A practicing physician with a sharp focus on finding the best methods to prevent and treat infections, Dr. Hall was a brilliant teacher, a supportive mentor, and a wife and mother known for her kind, gentle nature, her gift for poetry and the ceramic arts, and an endearing aptitude for fun.

Dr. Hall was an elected member of both the Institute of Medicine (now the National Academy of Medicine of the National Academy of Sciences) and the Royal College of Physicians. A founding member of the Pediatric Infectious Diseases Society, she served as its fifth president and historian. She chaired the American Academy of Pediatrics Committee on Infectious Diseases (Red Book Committee), whose 2006 edition was dedicated to her. She was a member of the Centers for Disease Control's Advisory Committee on Immunization Practices, of the Board of Scientific Counselors for the National Center of Infectious Diseases, and the American Board of Pediatrics.

Her many honors include the AAP's award for Lifetime Contribution to Infectious Diseases Education, the Distinguished Service Award from the Pediatric Infectious Diseases Society, the Infectious Diseases Society of America's John Franklin Enders Lectureship, the Pan American Society of

Virology's Award, and the Robert M. Chanock Lifetime Achievement Award named for the eminent virologist.

Caren Hall's name will be forever linked with that of her father, Burtis Burr Breese, MD, a distinguished physician/scientist with a specialty in meningo-coccal and streptococcal infections. A graduate of Harvard, Princeton, and Johns Hopkins, Dr. Breese co-founded Rochester's Elmwood Pediatric Group with two intentions: to treat children and to use his practice to conduct research on childhood infections. (He is credited with being the first to cul-ture "strep throat" in an office setting, using parts of a commercial incubator designed to hatch chicken eggs.)

"Professionally, Burr was an enormous influence on Caren," says her hus-band William J. Hall, MD, UR professor of medicine. He explains that Caren was infused with the spirit of medical research from an early age; Dr. Breese had a small laboratory behind the family's garage and another at their lakeside cottage in northern Michigan. As for teaching his daughter how to take care of patients, Dr. Breese had that well in hand, too. In those days, doctors made "house calls." "I'm going out to see a patient," Dr. Breese would say. "Come with me, Caren. You can drive." The teenager jumped at the invitation, and the bond strengthened.

A graduate of Rochester's Brighton High School, Wellesley College, and the University of Rochester School of Medicine and Dentistry, Caren was in the sec-ond year of her residency in pediatrics at Yale University when she was asked to supervise a group of first-year residents, all men. Among them was Bill Hall, a graduate of the University of Michigan, who was enrolled in a new medicine/ pediatric residency program being introduced at Yale's medical school.

Hall, a budding internist, was surprised on arrival to learn that pediatrics would be the group's first course of study. The chairman reassured the all-male group: "Don't worry, you have backup. I'm assigning a second-year resident who will countersign all your orders." The resident was brilliant, blonde, and beautiful. After a six-month whirlwind courtship, Dr. Caroline Breese and Dr. William Hall married in a simple ceremony in the living room of one of their professors. ("She countersigned my orders over the next forty years," says Dr. Hall, with loving regret for his now absent partner.)

Following residency, Caren traveled to Japan with Bill, who had been assigned there for military service. His "dream job": working with a research team in Hiroshima, investigating the effects on the population of radiation exposure from the atomic blast. Caren began a surveillance program on respiratory disease in local children, an effort her husband describes as an important part of her development as an epidemiologist/virologist. The couple's first child, a daughter, was born during those two years overseas.

Both Caren and Bill joined the UR faculty in 1971, with Caren originally hired by the Department of Medicine. At a time when knowledge of viruses was new and rapidly expanding, the cell-culture methods that Caren had learned at Yale were important. Few pediatric pathogens escaped her focus. Her investigations had widespread impact. The nasal washes she began taking from children were very successful in revealing RSV; her report on the incidence of RSV in neonates hospitalized for more than six days revealed that 50 percent of the infants' families also were infected. As a result of studies such as these, hundreds of her papers were published, including several in the prestigious *New England Journal of Medicine*.

Toward the end of her career, Dr. Hall began investigating how chromosomally inherited HHV-6 might affect intellectual function. That work was the basis for one of many papers published after her death.

The fact that Dr. Hall seemed blessed with a sunny, upbeat nature made her a favorite with students, faculty, and peers throughout her career. She sang and danced in medical center "follies" and she once brought to a party a piñata she had fashioned in the form of a streptococcus. As one former trainee said,

"If you were fortunate enough to be [Caren's] mentee, you were always front and center, the most important person in the room."

At home, medical science continued to be a presence for both Caren and her husband, Bill, also a distinguished faculty member at UR and former president of the American College of Physicians. Together they raised three children, helped by a series of daytime nannies. Daughter Kellyann is an attorney in San Francisco; son Burr is a cardiologist specializing in electrophysiology at Strong Memorial Hospital; and daughter Amity is a physician's assistant at Stanford University.

At a posthumous conference at the University that brought together Dr. Hall's colleagues, mentees, family, and friends from across the country, Dr. Peter Szilagyi spoke warmly on Dr. Hall's impact: "Caren had a profound influence on all of us who knew her. She had three great gifts. First, was her pure love of science. An incredible clinician, she was able to untangle complex clinical components to get the right diagnosis. The second was her power to use written and spoken language in ways in which each perfect phrase coalesced into a whole. The third was her gift from the heart, as shown by her many quiet acts of kindness." Dr. Caroline Hall was, indeed, a woman who will be long remembered.

Note

1. This profile was made possible thanks to help from William J. Hall, MD, Dr. Caroline Hall's husband.

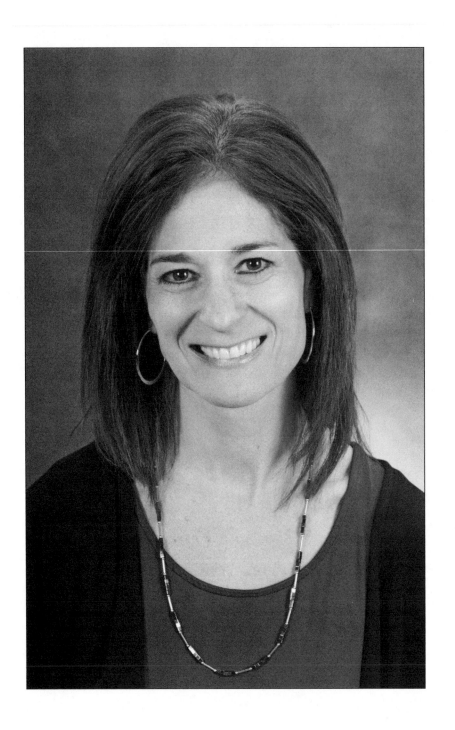

Chapter Sixteen

JILL S. HALTERMAN, MD, MPH

Dr. Jill Halterman holds several professional titles. Ask her what she does, and she makes it sound simple: "I care for patients in our primary clinic, I'm a physician-scientist who is investigating how best to deliver medical services to the underserved, specifically to children with asthma. I also serve as executive vice chair of the URMC Department of Pediatrics."

There is simply no way to translate that matter-of-fact statement into hours in the work week. Nor does it highlight the fact that Dr. Halterman leads one of the Department of Pediatrics's busiest NIH-funded clinical research laboratories, where fourteen full-time research assistants are working to determine the best ways to relieve the symptoms of asthma that keep so many inner-city children away from school and that often cause emergency visits or admissions to the hospital.

"We are investigating new models for bringing medical care to traditionally underserved children," she says. "Rochester is a perfect city for this kind of research because of the collaborations that have been built over time. Unfortunately, we see children who face many challenges, including suboptimal access to healthcare." Her community-based work is heavily supported by more than $10 million in NIH grants.

Halterman and her work get high praise from Dr. Elizabeth McAnarney, chair emerita of the Department of Pediatrics, who calls Jill's school-based, community approach to childhood asthma work of high national significance. "Jill is a unique individual possessing keen intellectual gifts, high personal integrity, energy, a delightful nature, and creativity applied consistently to all she undertakes. She is a role model for attaining work-life balance at a very high level."

A native of Penfield, New York, Jill grew up in a home where medical care for children was an everyday topic. Her father, Dr. George Segel, is a pediatric hematologist/oncologist. "My father is an amazing role model for how to truly care for patients," she says. "Although he was always very busy, he never viewed his career as a burden and would answer evening calls and work weekends as needed without ever suggesting it was an imposition." From him, she developed an understanding of the dedication that accompanies good patient care and learned to love the science behind medicine.

Jill's academic education is almost completely "all-Rochester," starting in nearby Penfield, where her high school record was stellar; she then attended the University of Rochester for her undergraduate work. Her performance in college was so outstanding that she was accepted into the UR's medical school as a sophomore. She received her bachelor's degree in 1990, graduating *summa cum laude* and Phi Beta Kappa with a specialty in psychology.

As a UR medical student, Jill knew early on that she was attracted to pediatrics as a career. "I saw working with children as a challenge that I would enjoy. I appreciate their resilience—and I looked forward to work that would allow me to engage with parents and caregivers," she says. Her undergraduate emphasis on psychology made her particularly interested in observing how children's minds develop. As a first-year medical student, she had the privilege of working with Dr. McAnarney, then chair of the department, on a study looking at the relationship between gestational weight gain and subsequent obesity in adolescent girls. "Jill's paper from that research has helped shape national medical care policy for adolescents," says McAnarney.

In 1994, Jill received her Doctor of Medicine Degree with honors. The ceremony was made more memorable by a special gift: Dr. Robert Hoekelman, former chair of pediatrics, presented Jill with her first neonatal stethoscope.

Later that year, Jill began her pediatric internship at Children's Hospital of Philadelphia, the only year she would spend away from her educational home in Rochester.

In 1995, Dr. Halterman came back home to Rochester to join her husband Marc, who was working on his MD/PhD degree, and to continue her postdoctoral training at Golisano Children's Hospital at Strong Memorial. She served first as an associate resident in pediatrics, and then as chief resident. In 1998, she began a three-year fellowship in general academic pediatrics, demanding work that soon led to her rise up the faculty appointments ladder. A clinical instructor at the start of her fellowship year, nine years later she was associate division chief and director of pediatric health services research for general pediatrics. In 2013, she became professor of pediatrics with unlimited tenure; in 2015, division chief in general pediatrics; and in 2018 she was named executive vice chair of the Department of Pediatrics.

Were there challenges along the way? A few, no doubt. Yet Jill says, "I never strayed far off my career path. My goals were fairly clear to me and I just went straight through." Meliora!

"I reached a decision point after my residency to focus my career on improving care for poor and underserved children," Dr. Halterman says. The best way to achieve that, she decided, was through general pediatrics. In recent years, her work has focused on a specific trouble point—asthma among underserved city children. In Rochester, more than 10 percent of urban children are affected, a rate substantially higher than for suburban children.

From that decision, two questions arose: What are the gaps in care for these children? And, what is the optimum way to deliver that care? "My early research explored barriers to guideline-based asthma care. We realized that there were gaps in the delivery of care at multiple levels," says Halterman. Her response: organizing a preventive care program for Rochester's urban children with asthma and a team to put the program into action. Team partners in the NIH-supported project include research investigators, program coordinators, nurses, research assistants, graduate and undergraduate medical students, and volunteers. Many of their programs are centered in the city schools, in order to reach children in the setting where they spend much of their day.

More than a decade ago, Halterman's team tested a model in partnership with the school nurse program that provided children with their preventive asthma medicine while they were at school. Thus, medication adherence could be assured on most days of the week. School nurses administer one daily dose of medication to each child. "It is exciting to see this is making a difference," says Halterman. Our greater goal is to develop sustainable models for asthma care that can be of use to physicians, caregivers, and healthcare researchers across the country. We are now seeing many other sites develop their own programs based on our work," Halterman says.

Dr. Halterman also serves as coach and mentor for dozens of young investigators. Many of her former mentees are now faculty members at medical centers across the country. Their interests are rich and varied, and many focus on how best to serve children in underserved urban or rural communities.

Dr. Marina Reznik, associate professor of pediatrics at Children's Hospital at Montefiore, was one of those trainees. "Jill has provided the most valuable and timely advice on my research and career development. She is not only an accomplished physician-scientist and leader, but also a caring colleague, friend, and role model," she says.

Dr. Halterman serves on multiple academic committees within the medical school, and she is an active reviewer for national and international professional journals. She is a member of the American Pediatric Society and the Society for Pediatric Research. She has received multiple awards for her leadership, teaching, and research.

How does a woman who wears so many hats—those of her professional roles as well as those of daughter, wife, and mother—manage such a full schedule? It's because she enjoys everything she does, she says. "I love working with my team, members of the division, and other investigators. We're all working together to achieve the same goals, and it is very rewarding. It also helps that I'm fairly efficient in my work and can get things done quickly. I also love my time away from work, particularly time with my family, and time to go to the gym to relieve stress!"

As mother of two teenagers, Halterman has tried to restrict the professional travel time she spends away from Rochester. Daughter Rebecca is a lively, active, high school student. Jill is a resolute mother, spending time with Rebecca each day to help her focus on homework. Son Justin is a UR biochemistry major. "He's a very serious and mature student," his mother says. "He has a scientific mind, so I suspect he will pursue a field of science in the future."

For those looking to enter the world of academic pediatrics, this high-achieving star has the following advice:

- Follow your passion.
- Focus on areas that are consistent with your strengths.
- Build and nurture effective teams.
- When making difficult decisions in your work, always keep patients and their families at the forefront.
- Keep a sense of humor!

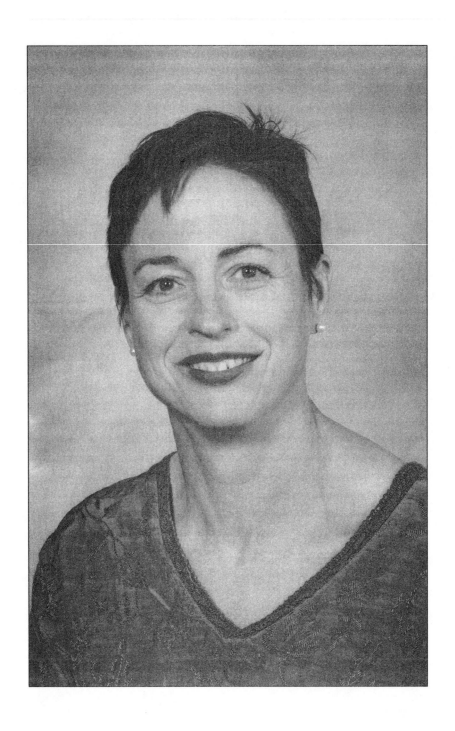

Chapter Seventeen

CYNTHIA R. HOWARD, MD, MPH

Back in the 1980s, Cindy Howard was a *really* busy young woman, trying to fit three big jobs into each twenty-four-hour day. At the Greenville Children's Hospital in South Carolina, she was working her way through her second year of residency in pediatrics. She was also building a life in a new part of the country with husband Fred, an obstetrician in private practice in Greenville. Perhaps most significantly, as a first-time mother, she was often sleep-deprived as she cared for their infant daughter.

During those first months of motherhood, you might have found Cindy with a diaper in one hand and a book in the other. In all probability, the book was *Breastfeeding*, by Dr. Ruth Lawrence, the University of Rochester pediatrician who was revolutionizing the way American women were feeding their infants.

Fast forward a decade and we find Dr. Cynthia Howard in Rochester working closely with Dr. Lawrence. Cindy had just been appointed director of the Rochester General Hospital (RGH) initiative to become a "baby-friendly hospital" and she was also directing its newborn nursery. "As a resident, I read Ruth's book cover to cover. For a while, it was my bible," Cindy says. What serendipity to be working closely—and unexpectedly—with the woman whose advice had guided her through her own first months as a mother.

David M. Siegel, MD, MPH, professor of pediatrics, chief of the Division of Pediatric Rheumatology, and chief of pediatrics at RGH, highly values what Dr. Howard has contributed over the years to the hospital's pediatric program:

Dr. Howard was already experienced in newborn care when she arrived in Rochester. She set about with meticulous technique and fierce advocacy to increase rates of breastfeeding among mothers delivering at our hospital. With patience, perseverance, and relentless focus, she succeeded in helping RGH become the first "baby-friendly hospital" in New York State and among the first in the country to be so designated by the World Health Organization (WHO). Cindy leaves an indelible legacy in our newborn nursery, where babies and mothers are beneficiaries of her pioneering work, as are the medical students and residents who train here.

It has been a long journey. For Cindy, as with several of her colleagues, finding financial resources for college was a challenge. Speaking of her school days in Denver, Colorado, she says, "I was a bright kid who benefited from the fact that Jefferson County schools had federal money to create enhanced science classes and to attract good, inspirational teachers. "This was the year of the first 'Earth Day,'" Cindy says, "and my long-term senior project involved collecting and analyzing water samples that we kids collected from local streams and rivers."

"I met my first mentor at that time," she says. "My dermatologist, Dr. Anna Loeffler, took an interest in three of us high school girls who all were interested in science. She was very supportive. She took us to meetings of the women's branch of the local medical society whenever the subject was careers in medicine. If I ever expressed doubts about my ability to go to college, she always stressed, 'You can do this!'"

Cindy did well as an undergraduate at the University of Colorado. She was strong in all her science classes and graduated in 1975 with a BA with an emphasis on microbiology. When the time came to consider the possibility of postgraduate studies, finances once again were the big issue. "My parents were children of the Depression," says Cindy. "I needed a career that could support me, but also enable me to help my mother and father as they grew older." She considered her options: Become a nurse-practitioner? Go to medical school? Get a PhD in microbiology? "I took the best offer and went to medical school," she says, with a big smile.

Dr. Howard received her medical degree from the University of Colorado Health Sciences Center in Denver in 1981. During a rotation at Denver's Children's Hospital, she chose her career focus: pediatrics. Working with the children, helping their parents, and learning from the residents, interns, and faculty, she thought, "I really like doing this!" The young woman who had expected to be a microbiologist discovered that she wanted to work not in a laboratory but with people.

Cindy was a senior in medical school in Denver when she met the man she would marry. As part of the Health Service Corps, Fred Howard was finishing his medical residency at Fitzsimons Army Medical Center in nearby Aurora. As it happened, Cindy was assigned to Fitzsimons for her obstetrics and gynecology senior student experience. "I had made a vow never to date anyone [I worked with] on service. I broke my own rule, though," she says with a smile. "I was engaged eight weeks later and married in five months." Fred, who was five years ahead of Cindy in training, soon became a major in the Army Medical Corps.

When Fred completed his military service at Fort Jackson, South Carolina, the couple needed to put down roots. Cindy finished her pediatric residency at the Greenville Health System Children's Hospital and Fred joined a private obstetrics and gynecology practice. Cindy became board-certified in pediatrics in 1987.

As with many young couples, money—including repayment of college loans—was an issue for the Howards. Physicians were scarce at that time in rural South Carolina, and Cindy realized here was an opportunity to apply for her first real job as a doctor while fulfilling her obligation to the National Health Services Scholarship program. She contacted several of the region's congressmen seeking support and offering them a deal that was hard to refuse. She would work as a traveling pediatrician for the state health department *without pay* if she could be assigned to cover a territory within ninety miles of the family's home in Greenville. A senator, she says, made that happen—and for the next four years, Dr. Cynthia Howard would drive 40,000 miles a year seeing patients at state-funded health clinics throughout the ten neighboring counties. (One of Dr. Howard's best memories of those traveling years is how she succeeded in arranging primary pediatric care for a number of children with complicated medical problems.)

Dr. Howard's clinical work for South Carolina's Upper Savannah Health District soon expanded, as she became, sequentially, medical director of the Children's Trust Fund Grant and the Breastfeeding Promotion Project. At the University of South Carolina School of Medicine, she was appointed a clinical instructor in 1990 and that same year she became director of the Newborn Nursery at Children's Hospital in Greenville. "That was a job I really loved," she says. "The nursery took care of six thousand newborns a year. I worked as director of the nursery and taught both Family Medicine and Pediatric residents."

In 1991, Fred and Cindy came to Rochester, where Fred was interviewing for a faculty post in Obstetrics and Gynecology. A high point in the trip came one evening when the couple went to meet Dr. Michael Weitzman, chief of pediatrics at Rochester General Hospital (RGH), who met the South Carolina couple at Hattie's, a popular cocktail bar. Fred was hired, and so was Cindy, as a senior instructor in Pediatrics, a fellow in general academic pediatrics, and, soon, director of RGH's newborn nursery.

Dr. Siegel points out that as director of the nursery, Cindy applied careful observation and research methodology to answering important questions regarding full-term babies. "She first identified the characterization and amelioration of pain associated with circumcision as an understudied area and gathered data making the case that newborns *do* experience pain and that the discomfort of a procedure can be effectively and safely addressed," he says.

Recalling those early days, Dr. Howard says, "Rochester is a wonderful place to raise a family, and I had a fabulous job, including teaching residents in the nursery. Both Pediatric department chair, Bob Hoekelman, and colleague Mike Weitzman strongly supported faculty independence. Bob knew I had a small child and very thoughtfully suggested I delay beginning work until September." She points out that RGH's relatively small Department of Pediatrics continues to promote a strong family feeling. "Not only have I made long-term friends, but I was able to get my Masters in Public Health [in 1997]."

Shortly after her arrival, Cindy connected with Dr. Ruth Lawrence, whose book on breastfeeding had so helped her as a new mother. In 1991 they wrote two commentaries that charted the degree to which manufacturers of "formula" were marketing their products through free samples in obstetrical and pediatric offices. That same year, Dr. Howard was first author on a clinical trial based on WHO "baby friendly" recommendations indicating that "best care" for the mother-baby dyad should include educational materials for expectant mothers that promote breastfeeding. (The baby-friendly hospital initiative is now the standard of care for participating hospitals throughout the world.)

In 1996, Dr. Howard became a charter member of the Academy of Breastfeeding Medicine (ABM), a multi-specialty organization focused on educating physicians on the nutritional and psychological importance of breastfeeding. In addition to being a past president of ABM, she is currently a senior advisor to the board of directors and has served in leading roles on all its committees.

At the state and national level, Dr. Howard has been active in all major organizations that support breastfeeding, including the International Society for Research in Human Milk and Lactation, La Leche International, the W. K. Kellogg Foundation, and the New York State Breastfeeding Coalition as well as the American Academy of Pediatrics.

Dr. Howard speaks glowingly of her years in Rochester, praising the academic environment as she has experienced it. "Years ago, I noticed in medical journals how many important papers came out of Rochester," she says. "I've loved being part of the mix of clinical care, teaching, and research. As technology advanced, I could work on my research in free hours at home."

The praise continues, especially for the general pediatrics program in which Dr. Howard built her career. "I was very fortunate to work here. We have chiefs who understand, who realize faculty have other lives—and that's very unusual nationally. We also can boast a long-standing career success rate for our graduates." As a woman who has been mentored by others—including her mother, "my first and best mentor"—Cindy has passed this gift on to her own mentees.

Recently retired, Dr. Howard continues her connection with URMC and with her colleagues in pediatrics across the country. She and Fred live in Rochester, but spend winter months on their sailboat in the Caribbean.

Dr. Howard shares the following frank advice for young people who choose a career in academic medicine:

- Figure out how to get protected time for your research. (Find a mentor who can help you negotiate that.)
- Find a niche or two that are important and where you can become the expert.
- Get enough balls in the air so that if some drop, others will be successful.
- Expect to get a paper out of every one of your grand rounds presentations. (You will have spent eighty to one hundred hours preparing. Don't waste the effort.)
- Get a review paper or the background for a grant prepared. As you work, figure out what's next to investigate. Then revamp the presentation, run it another way, and present the material in a different form to a different audience.
- Never work part-time. (You'll be paid part-time, but you'll work full-time anyway.)
- Build your reputation as an expert.
- Get involved in relevant organizations. They are often key to advocacy around important children's issues.

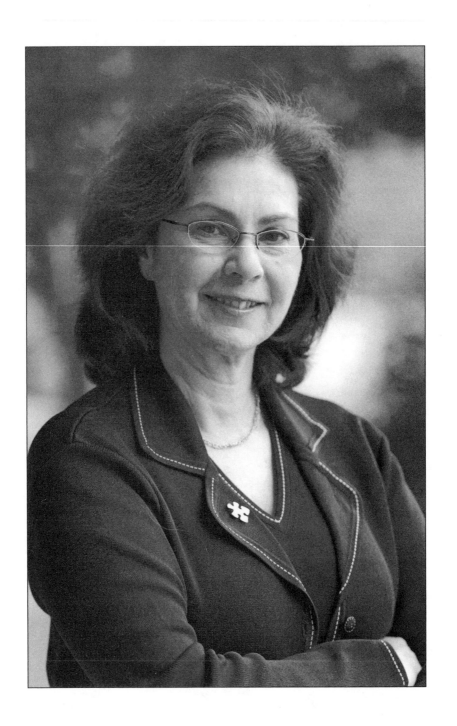

Chapter Eighteen

SUSAN L. HYMAN, MD

Dr. Susan Hyman is one of the country's leading advocates for patients and families who are facing the challenge of living with autism. In the mid-1990s, Hyman was one of a small group of investigators whose research propelled the University of Rochester into the national autism conversation. Since then, her passion for patients has extended far beyond the clinic and laboratory. Her goal: to develop and promote a model medical environment where patients and families can easily access the multiple resources that living with autism requires and then to share that model with other healthcare communities.

As chair of the subcommittee on autism of the American Academy of Pediatrics from its inception until 2014, and now as a member of the Executive Committee on Children with Disabilities, Dr. Hyman brings three decades of treatment and research to a condition that confronts millions of families. Her public profile notes that she is no stranger to controversy. She has challenged the notion of a link between vaccines and autism in the national media. She has also questioned the effectiveness of popular gluten- and casein-free diets for those with autism, her skepticism being grounded in evidence-based research.

These days, Dr. Hyman leads the Division of Developmental and Behavioral Pediatrics, one of the Department of Pediatrics's largest divisions and home to one of twelve Autism Speaks Autism Treatment Network centers across the US and Canada. "With twenty-six faculty and more than sixty staff, our division is a microcosm of the whole Department of Pediatrics," she says. "My job as chief is to weave into this tapestry all the strands of our many-colored mission."

Susan Hyman grew up in Suffern, New York, in a family environment that was very supportive of her choice of medicine as a career. Her father, a dermatologist, was health commissioner for Rockland County. Her brother is an internist, and now two of her nephews are physicians. At Brown University, where Hyman took both her undergraduate and medical degrees, fully half of her medical school classmates were women and the dean's wife was a pathologist. "I grew up with women who were doctors," she says. It's a world Dr. Hyman knows well.

"I entered medical school thinking I would go into public health, because I was influenced by seeing my father make community health decisions," she says. "I did not enjoy my clinical rotations until I came to pediatrics, which immediately I loved." The choice became clear. Dr. Hyman completed her pediatric residency at North Carolina Memorial Hospital in Chapel Hill. Her next career choice emerged from an assignment in the spina bifida clinic. "That experience changed my whole focus," she says. "The children and families were wonderful, and clinically I was involved with challenging and interesting cognitive disorders. Perhaps the most important lesson I learned at that clinic was this: 'We might not be able to cure children with developmental disorders, but we could make life better.'"

After her residency, she pursued fellowship training in developmental disabilities at the Kennedy-Kreiger Institute at Johns Hopkins Hospital in Baltimore. She says her program director, Dr. Arnold Capute, founder of neurodevelopmental disabilities as a subspecialty field, was notorious for giving his female fellows a rough time. Years later when Dr. Hyman was awarded the Arnold Capute Award by the Council on Children with Disabilities of the American Academy of Pediatrics, she said of Dr. Capute, "Those were the days when Arnold felt men were men and girls were girls, until they became his fellows."

Hyman's first academic position was as an attending physician at Hopkins. In 1985, she was appointed director of the Self-Injurious Behavior Unit at Kennedy-Kreiger Institute. This inpatient setting provided intense behavioral interventions for children and youth with autism and intellectual difficulties. Her clinical work was complemented by collaboration in research investigating a newly described disorder, Rett Syndrome. She continued collaborating in this research when she assumed her second academic position at the University of Maryland in the Maternal Child Health Bureau-funded Developmental and Behavioral Pediatrics program. This outpatient position was more conducive to raising her two young children.

The traffic jam on the congested Beltway around Washington, DC, was the catalyst that brought Dr. Hyman and her physician husband, Dr. William Fricke, to Rochester in the early 1990s. "Bill was working then at the FDA in Bethesda. One day, stuck in the usual early-morning gridlock, he had an epiphany. He said, 'Let's go someplace where there's no traffic.'" Rochester's Genesee Hospital needed a hematopathologist, so Bill, Susan, and their preschoolers moved north. Susan worked first two, then three, days a week as an assistant professor at the Strong Center for Developmental Disabilities, a precursor to the current division.

It was a good move. At that time, working quietly in her UR laboratory, Dr. Patricia Rodier was putting together clues on how genes in the developing brain seemed to be associated with the developmental risk for autism. A brilliant embryologist, Rodier was among the first cohort of women scientists, doing groundbreaking research and working alone, as many basic scientists did in those days. Rodier needed a clinical researcher to help prove her hypotheses linking early developmental genes regulating brain development to the occurrence of autism. In a proverbial quirk of fate (praise for Hyman from a colleague to Rodier during a break at an NIH state of the science meeting on autism), Susan became Rodier's research partner.

As a result of Rodier's research, Rochester would soon burst onto the national map as a leader in autism research. "Within a year, we had an RO1 grant, and then a larger Collaborative Program in Excellence (CPEA) and then a second program project grant, Studies to Advance Autism Research in Treatment (STAART)," says Dr. Hyman. "With that, we jumped immediately from the minor league to the majors, and with the leadership of our research group by Tristram Smith, PhD, we have remained a powerhouse. We're at another critical moment now, as we consider ways to intervene and improve brain function, not just for autism but other neurodevelopmental disorders."

As chief of her division, Dr. Hyman's multiple roles now include supporting young investigators and mid-career faculty. "Nothing in my medical training prepared me for this leadership position," she says. "I've had multiple twists and turns in my career. Fortunately, I've learned to refocus myself to meet each new challenge."

For her own leadership training, Dr. Hyman found exceptional support from colleagues in the AAP. She is also very grateful that the University of Rochester nominated her and fostered her participation in a year-long Executive Leadership in Academic Medicine program (ELAM) for women in academic medicine sponsored by Drexel University. Working on issues at both the local and national levels is now a big part of her career. As the American Academy of Pediatrics meets the challenges of a changing world, Hyman is playing a major role preparing for the future, helping set policy for screening guidelines and medical care for children and youth with autism spectrum disorders in the medical home.

This work is complemented by her work with the Autism Speaks Autism Treatment Network that is setting the standards for clinical diagnosis and care of children with autism spectrum disorders and developing strategies for the standards' widespread dissemination. The Autism Speaks Autism Treatment Network supported Dr. Hyman's research on diet, nutrition, and feeding behavior in autism. The national registry of seven thousand patients, including patients from Rochester, has been instrumental in documenting a possible correlation between anxiety and gastrointestinal problems in patients with autism spectrum disorders, as well as descriptive data on other co-occurring conditions.

Dr. Hyman is active in several national and local organizations that focus on the needs of children and youth with developmental disabilities. In addition to serving on the Executive Committee of the Council of

Children with Disabilities and the Autism Subcommittee of the American Academy of Pediatrics, she is on the Scientific Advisory Board of the Autism Science Foundation and locally is a board member of Autism Up and the Autism Family Center. Her professional memberships include the Society for Developmental and Behavioral Pediatrics, the American Academy of Cerebral Palsy and Developmental Medicine, and the International Society for Autism Research.

The Rochester site of the Autism Treatment Network is collaborating in an innovative telementoring program designed to test the ECHO model for supporting the medical home in the care of children with autism spectrum disorders as an example of a complex chronic condition. "I'm very excited about this work," she says. "The ECHO model uses technology to create an interactive community of primary care providers with a team at the UR Medical Center. Brief didactic sessions are complemented with discussion of real cases the primary care providers are working with." Dr. Hyman is also lead author of *The AAP Autism Tool Kit*, a manual that provides clinical information for community physicians to care for children with autism.

Clinically, Dr. Hyman is an attending pediatrician at Golisano Children's Hospital and at Monroe Community Hospital. She sees outpatients through the clinical services of the Division of Developmental and Behavioral Pediatrics and Levine Autism Clinic.

Dr. Hyman and her husband, Dr. William Fricke, have two adult children. Their daughter graduated from Washington University in St. Louis, Missouri, and their son from the University of Rochester. Both are currently pursuing graduate degrees.

The following counsel for young women considering a career in medicine has been mined from Dr. Hyman's long and varied career:

- Medicine isn't a job with hour limits. Your work doesn't end at five o'clock. Neither does your job as a doctor or as a spouse and parent.
- Choose a career path that fits your passion and your personality.

- As you build your career, be nimble and have foresight. Watch for what's trending; not just in science, but within the system where you are working.
- Read Sheryl Sandberg's book, *Lean In: Women, Work, and the Will to Lead*.
- Find a "sisterhood" within your professional organizations.
- Take time now and then to reflect on where you want to go. Then listen to yourself.
- You'll have to work for success, both at work and at home. Don't expect to be given it.
- Above all, believe in yourself.

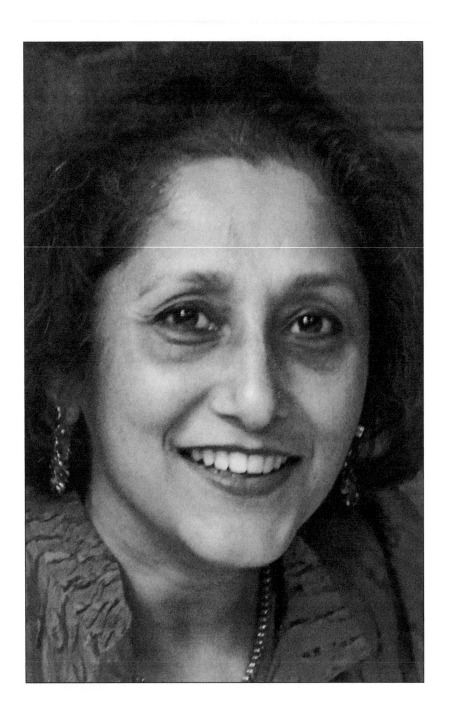

Chapter Nineteen

NIRUPAMA B. LAROIA, MBBS, MD

Dr. Nirupama Laroia thinks big. Her mission is global: teaching healthcare providers in rural or underserved communities how to save the lives of newborns struggling for breath by using inexpensive, low-tech resuscitation tools. Imagine a mother giving birth in a primary healthcare center in rural India. Her infant gasps, struggles in vain to breathe. Quickly, the attending midwife places a tiny mask over the newborn's face and manually pumps life-saving air into the tiny lungs from a bag attached to the mask. A minute later, the baby's first cry is heard.

"In the western world, medicine has advanced so far that it's rare to have full-term babies die because they can't breathe," says Dr. Laroia. "That's not true for the rest of the world. Simple life-saving measures can save many of these babies. Our challenge is to teach those present at the birth how to use simple tools that are effective even when electricity and other technological resources are absent." Currently, Laroia has expanded her effort to include understanding and promoting ways to improve healthcare for immigrant mothers and their infants in the US.

Dr. Laroia's workshops, classes, and training sessions for UR medical students and fellows spread the message, and her call to action resonates through the national pediatrics community. National boundaries are no hindrance to Laroia, who often moderates neonatology conferences in her native India. Each August, she spends three weeks in remote villages high in the Himalayas, teaching nurses, midwives, and doctors at the district hospital and primary health centers how to resuscitate and care for newborns. She works alongside Dr. Nancy Chin, an anthropologist and a colleague in Public Health Sciences who joins her in researching the social determinants of health in isolated mountain villages.

Dr. Laroia's professional links include memberships in the American Academy of Pediatrics; the Eastern Society for Pediatric Research (ESPR); the Indian Academy of Pediatrics; and India's National Neonatology Forum.

Nirupama Laroia was born in India into a family with a strong medical tradition. Her father, a US-trained radiologist, was a medical pioneer during the early 1950s, years when India was newly independent. Her grandfather, also a doctor, served in the Indian army before independence and continued to practice in his hometown into his eighth decade. Her husband is an obstetrician-gynecologist.

Her childhood home is abundant with accomplished women. Her mother, now retired, was a professor of political science at the women's college of Delhi University. Of Nirupama's three sisters, one has a PhD in psychology, specializing in juvenile forensic psychology; another, with a PhD in nutrition, works with the United Nations World Food Program; the third has an MBA and works for a pharmaceutical company.

"Going to university was an expectation for all of us," Nirupama says. In 1980, she received her bachelor of medicine bachelor of surgery degree (MBBS, the equivalent of an MD in countries that follow the UK system of education) from Christian Medical College in Ludhiana, Punjab, where she started her postgraduate training in obstetrics and gynecology. She changed her mind and completed her residency training in pediatrics from the Institute of Medical Sciences of Banaras Hindu University in Varanasi, following which she served as senior resident at Ram Manohar Lohia Hospital in New Delhi. While in medical school she met Rahul Laroia, and they married soon after she graduated from medical school.

Nirupama knew early on that she wanted to be a pediatrician and save newborns who have breathing problems. During her residency in pediatrics, news had spread about a miracle intervention—the use of surfactant—that was saving the lives of thousands of newborns in England and in the US. But surfactant therapy was far beyond the reach of India's medical community. To complete training in their specialties, the young couple—with their two young sons (the youngest just five weeks old)—left India for England.

Two years later, after her sons had grown beyond babyhood, Nirupama resumed her medical training and began rotating through various hospitals, as required by Britain's medical educational system. Over the next four years, Dr. Laroia was senior house officer in pediatrics at hospitals in Salisbury and Lincoln; in community health and pediatrics in Lincoln; and in neonatology at London's Hammersmith Hospital, where she did most of her neonatology training. She continued with her neonatology rotation at Leicester General Hospital and her general pediatrics training at Leicester's Royal Infirmary. Her last United Kingdom posting was as registrar at Walsgrave Hospital in Coventry.

"After all that moving around, both my husband and I were ready to settle down," she says. "Settling down" meant another move, this time across the Atlantic to the Medical College of Virginia in Richmond, where Nirupama began a fellowship in neonatal-perinatal medicine, investigating neonatal seizures from birth-related asphyxia. There she learned to use electroencephalography to track seizure patterns in neonates.

Postings in rural health centers both in India and in England strengthened her resolve to focus on effective ways to teach those attending births how to prevent asphyxia. "A baby's first breath is critical," she says. "There should always be someone in attendance who knows how to assist a newborn baby using a simple 'breath bag' to force air into tiny lungs and how to effectively resuscitate a frail newborn." "Training the trainer" has become one of Dr. Laroia's principal teaching efforts.

In 1994, Nirupama joined UR Pediatrics as a neonatology fellow under the leadership of Dr. Dale Phelps, and she completed the second two years of her neonatal-perinatal fellowship in Rochester. The opportunity enabled Dr.

Laroia to rejoin her husband, who had joined Rochester General Hospital to continue his residency training in the US. In 1997, a second fellowship in experimental therapeutics introduced her to UR's Clinical Trials Coordination Center, where she learned to conduct clinical trials.

She joined the neonatology faculty in 1996 as a senior instructor, and advanced to professor of pediatrics, the position she now holds. Since 1999, she has been the medical director of the Special Care Nursery and section chief of neonatology at Rochester General Hospital.

Supporting the local community is also important to Dr. Laroia. She is especially proud of her work on the board of Daystar for Medically Fragile Children, the state's only pediatric respite center for families with medically fragile children. At Daystar, pediatric nurses, therapists, and early education teachers provide skilled care for infants and children as they transition from hospital to home and allow parents to go back to work. This family-support effort, an outreach of the Sisters of St. Joseph, is available until the child enters kindergarten.

Among Laroia's many teaching roles, a highlight is her leading role in RGH's annual Townsend Teaching Day, a memorial event named in honor of Dr. Edward Townsend, Jr. (chief of pediatrics at Rochester General Hospital from 1956–65) that brings together national and local neonatologists, community physicians, and nurses who explore a broad range of topics common to every-day practice, including those relating to neonatology, obstetrics, surgery, and professionalism.

Over the years, Dr. Laroia has been helped by several mentors. "My mother was a great role model," she says. "Growing up in India, I saw her face gender differences head on and not be thwarted by them." At Hammersmith Hospital in London, Laroia's department chief helped channel her research by insisting she focus on questions that can have an answer. On her arrival in Rochester, Dr. Dale Phelps, the division chief, "helped me think a question through to its conclusion, while avoiding the mistake of assuming what I might find." Dr. Ronnie Guillet and Dr. Margaret McBride mentored her work with neonatal seizures and electroencephalography. Dr. Nancy Chin introduced her to the social sciences and taught her to respect qualitative research and ethnographic work.

Young women who envision a life that combines career and family can learn much from Dr. Laroia, a woman who has not only "walked the walk," but also raised two children on three continents while working. Son Gaurav is a lawyer in Washington, DC, who works as Policy Counsel with Free Press, an independent "government watchdog body." Son Asheesh is a software engineer, passionate about open-source software, and currently works in San Francisco.

"Finding the balance between work and family is a challenge," Nirupama admits, "one I couldn't have met without great help from my husband. It's also an interesting journey during which you learn a lot about yourself." Nirupama also advises women who want to pursue a career in medicine to:

- Find your focus, and then let your passion guide you along the way.
- You can't do everything every day. Learn to balance work, life, and family by scheduling responsibilities at different times throughout the week.
- Every job has its challenges. Meet yours one at a time.
- Envision your life as an evolving process, one that requires time and patience.

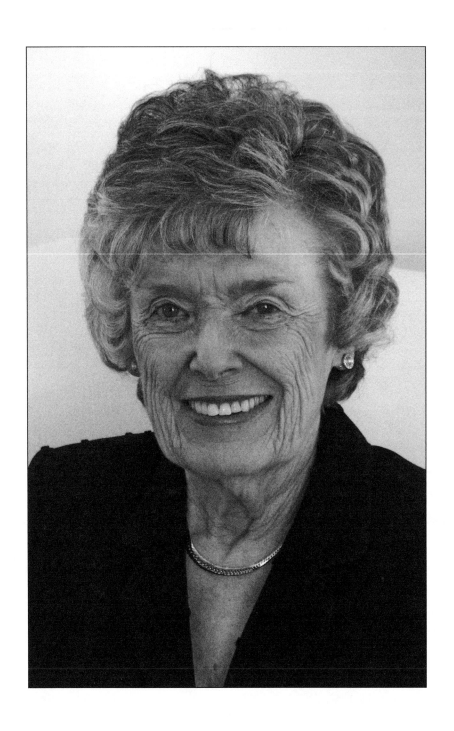

Chapter Twenty

RUTH A. LAWRENCE, MD

In 1978, a young associate professor at the University of Rochester School of Medicine and Dentistry began writing a book. Even though her days were busy—she was a clinician, a teacher, and a researcher—she was determined to snatch a few nighttime hours typing at home, while her children were asleep.

When Dr. Ruth Lawrence's book—*Breastfeeding: A Guide for the Medical Professional*—was published in 1980, it was a salvo that would change the culture of how American mothers nurtured their children. Lawrence's research on the benefits of breastfeeding for both mother and child helped shift the pattern away from families using commercially produced infant nutrition, commonly called "formula," to a "natural" model, with mother as loving provider.

Now in its eighth edition and translated into three languages, *Breastfeeding* not only changed the culture of baby care, it made Ruth Lawrence an internationally known lactation expert. Now in her ninth decade, Dr. Lawrence is still busy as an author, lecturer, teacher, mentor, researcher, mother (of nine), and grandmother.

What kind of young woman would turn down a four-year, all-expenses-paid scholarship to Radcliffe College, "sister school" to Harvard University? Begin by realizing that here is a woman confident enough to chart her own path. For Ruth Anderson, that early path was full of stumbling blocks shaped by the Great Depression. Ruth's widowed mother, once well-to-do, was forced to move her little family fourteen times during Ruth's teenage years.

"We had nothing. We just did the best we could," says Dr. Lawrence about those hard times. To see the family through, Ruth's mother played the organ at church weddings; she also taught tennis at the private Scarborough School in Briarcliff Manor, set among the grand estates of New York's Westchester County. A scholarship student at Scarborough, young Ruth relished her classes in science and math; at home, she was often responsible for cooking and taking care of her younger sister and brother. "Mother never let us think we were poor, but I learned that life could be hard—and that I would have to test myself," she says. (The painful thought of living among stylish undergraduate Radcliffe students led her to decide not to attend.)

In 1941, a major scholarship from a Manhattan foundation and a clutch of prizes enabled Ruth to travel west to Antioch College, a highly rated liberal arts college that ranked among the country's ten best small colleges. "At Antioch, I learned to be a contributing person," says Dr. Lawrence. Four years later, she would graduate *summa cum laude* with distinction in biology and a strong interest in physics. Except for her scholarships, "I went to college on my own nickel," Dr. Lawrence says proudly. She worked in the college cafeteria, which enabled her to get to know everyone on campus. (A required class in personal finance required students to prepare a personal financial statement. When the professor looked through Ruth's budget, he said, "You can't live on this!" Her response: "Watch me!")

With World War II raging, a required co-op job working in the lubricant laboratory at the Chrysler plant in Detroit made one thing clear: "After working week after week with oil and grease, I thought, if this is what physics is like, I'm going back to campus and changing my major," Dr. Lawrence recalls. The next summer found her heading to Chicago for a job at a co-op store in Hyde Park. A job, yes, but she had no place to stay—until she was welcomed as a "house sitter" by a woman pediatrician with a private practice, who was often away at a lake house. Dr. Vida Wentz told young Ruth: "If you work hard, you'll get where you want to go." It was a lesson she already knew by heart.

Next came a *real* Antioch co-op job: working in the medical library of CIBA Pharmaceutical Company in Summit, New Jersey, where company president Ernst Oppenheimer supported a student intern program. After talking with

Ruth, Dr. "Op" soon changed her job description; he sent her to CIBA's animal research laboratories where the first physiological tests were being made on the effects of antihistamines.

With continuing help from another influential mentor, Antioch's chair of biology, Ruth was awarded a summer scholarship at a private research laboratory, chief source of the world's supply of purebred mice, in Bar Harbor, Maine. "It was marvelous," she recalls. "I graduated from Antioch looking for a summer job and was awarded a summer research experience with all expenses paid. We lived in tents in woods surrounding the lab and did basic science research. I studied the lymphoid patches in the intestines of hamsters."

With a curriculum vitae that now included citations of work from two major laboratories and a distinguished college record, Ruth was accepted at the University of Rochester School of Medicine and Dentistry. Prior to admission, she had received a handwritten note from Dr. George Whipple, founding dean of UR's medical school, urging her to come to Rochester for an interview; he wrote, "Time and money should be no object." Ruth took the train north, and met with Dean Whipple; with Dr. William L. Bradford, the school's second chair of pediatrics; and with the chair of anatomy (a man less than enthusiastic about accepting a woman candidate). "I interviewed and was accepted six weeks later. A second note from Dr. Whipple read: "Congratulations. You have a seat in the Class entering in 1945."

When Ruth arrived in Rochester, a solidly founded and rapidly growing program in pediatrics, then entering its third decade, was a hallmark of the UR medical school. Quiet, scholarly Dr. Samuel W. Clausen, first chair of pediatrics, had been chosen by Dean Whipple as one of the ten original faculty. A fine teacher and an active researcher (co-identifier of fatty oil as the agent in "peanut bronchitis"), Clausen also maintained an active, informal relationship with students, aided by his wife, Edith, a British-born scientist.

Gender differences then were obvious: Of the sixty-five students in Ruth's class, for the first time thirteen were women. That gain was brief; World War II ended in August 1945.

Ruth's medical school days were notable for a very personal reason: she met Robert "Bob" Lawrence, a fellow student planning a career as a surgeon. Four years later, on Match Day, 1949, the young sweethearts discovered they would be spending their internship year apart: Ruth at Yale University and Bob at the University of Rochester.

At Yale, a life-changing experience for Ruth began in 1951 when she was awarded a fellowship year working with Yale pediatrician and psychiatrist Dr. Edith Jackson, then revolutionizing the model of infant care. Dr. Jackson had introduced the concept of "rooming-in," putting mothers together with their newborn infants, at Grace-New Haven Hospital. She actively promoted breastfeeding as important physically and psychologically for both mother and baby, and her article in the *Journal of the American Medical Association*, "Management of Breastfeeding," circulated widely throughout the nation's birthing centers. The movement was gaining increasing popular support.

As both a fellow and resident, Ruth worked on the Rooming-In Project at Grace-New Haven, and her work with Dr. Jackson continued during her term as chief resident in the newborn service at Yale New Haven Hospital. "The Jackson Experience" would forever help shape Ruth's own impressive career.

The Korean War interrupted life for Ruth and her surgeon sweetheart. When Bob was suddenly called to report for active duty in 1951, the young doctors decided to marry immediately. Returning to Ruth's home in Dutchess County, New York, they wed at the little chapel in Hyde Park, a ceremony graced by a bouquet whose blooms had been "borrowed" from the nearby gardens at President Franklin D. Roosevelt's family home. For the first six months of the following year, after Bob returned from Korea, Dr. Ruth Lawrence was a consultant in medicine at the Army hospital at Fort Dix, New Jersey. In Korea, Bob served in the legendary MASH (mobile army surgical hospital) unit. As a result of that horrific experience, he would change his specialty from surgery to anesthesiology.

In 1952, when Bob's military service ended, the Lawrences returned to Rochester, where Ruth became both a clinical instructor in pediatrics and a research pediatrician in the Monroe County Health Department, then led by the influential Dr. Albert Kaiser. Over the next decades, a series of career advances would include senior instructor in pediatrics, chief of the nursery service at Strong Memorial Hospital, and chief of pediatrics at Highland Hospital.

Dr. Lawrence's state- and nationwide role in poison control efforts during the mid-century years matches her work as a lactation expert. The field was opened to Lawrence by Dr. William Bradford who, in 1959, appointed her medical director of the Finger Lakes Regional Poison and Drug Information Center, the second of its kind in the nation and the first to take calls from the public, initiating a new concept in medical emergency services.

From her office at Strong Memorial Hospital (and at home, where her phone had a fifty-foot long cord), Ruth or someone on her small staff answered phone calls from the public—a mother whose child had swallowed a cleaning product, an adult with eyes affected by a possibly toxic substance, or a worried mushroom-gatherer—and provided callers with answers from toxicologists.

Dr. Lawrence was soon on the road, spending what would become thousands of hours promoting the service at schools, Parent Teacher Association (PTA) meetings, and corporate offices, distributing educational materials—and encouraging the growth of such centers across the country. In 1982, she presented the results of her Poison Center research at the International Congress of Clinical Toxicology at Snowmass, Colorado, and later served a two-year term as president of New York State's Poison Centers. (In 2010, Rochester's Poison Center was closed, a victim of state budget-cutting.)

In 1985, Dr. Lawrence was appointed founding director of the UR's Breastfeeding and Human Lactation Center. Nationally, she has chaired the breastfeeding section of the American Academy of Pediatrics and over the years has been a major contributor to summit meetings on the topic in Washington, DC, sponsored by the Kellogg Foundation. Founding editor of the journal *Breastfeeding Medicine*, her publications include 173 first-author citations; further, she is named in dozens of abstracts and journal reviews.

Dr. Lawrence's work as a breastfeeding advocate has taken her around the world, visits often paired with each new translation of her classic textbook. Most important to her personally, was her audience with Pope John Paul II in 1995, during which she urged the Pope to encourage women of the world to breastfeed.

As a consultant, she has served the Joseph P. Kennedy, Jr. Foundation, the Robert Wood Johnson Foundation, the Food and Drug Administration (FDA), Cornell University, Columbia University, the State of New York, and others. Within the Rochester community, she has served as board chairman for Monroe Community Hospital and the Safety Council.

Of her many awards, Dr. Lawrence is particularly proud that the poison center she founded bore her name, that Antioch College honored her with the Horace Mann Medal for her contribution to mankind, and that she holds an honorary Doctor of Divinity degree from St. Bernard's Institute in Rochester.

Ruth Lawrence has much to say that is relevant for young women entering medicine. The key to being a good doctor, Dr. Lawrence insists, is to really care about your patient. The science will come and go, but the best doctors understand people, real people, and are good communicators. Listen when patients talk, listen completely.

Other advice from one who has done it all:

- Family first! (If you plan on getting married, make sure you and your partner have the same goals and beliefs. I was lucky to find the best man in the world.)
- If you're ambitious, be ready to jump through the hoops. A Doctor of Medicine (MD) degree probably won't be enough. Pick a specialty.

- Don't let them see you sweat! We women have to stop making excuses for ourselves.

As for "the good old days" of the 1950s, she says, "Honestly, we women were not welcome [in medicine]. Often, I never was paid for much of the work I was doing. At the time, I was just glad to be taking responsibility for the hospital nursery. I seized that opportunity and, in the process, helped pioneer neonatology as a specialty—and eventually became a world authority on the benefits of breastfeeding."

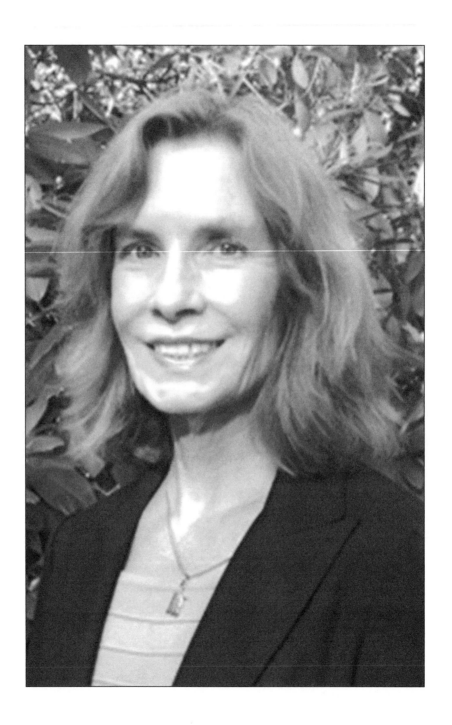

Chapter Twenty-One

ANN M. LENANE, MD

Today, at midcareer, Dr. Ann Lenane is deeply involved in one of medicine's most emotionally challenging fields: evaluating and managing care for children subjected to often horrific abuse. Dr. Lenane is one of only a relatively few physicians in the nation board-certified in the field of child abuse pediatrics.

As medical director of the Department of Pediatrics's program for Referral and Evaluation for Abused Children (REACH), Dr. Lenane focuses her work on the young victims of abuse and their families as well as interacting with the many professionals involved in the evaluation and treatment of child abuse: Child Protective Service (CPS) caseworkers, social workers, police investigators, attorneys, family advocates, and counselors. Key to the medical evaluation of suspected child abuse is Dr. Lenane's link with other specialist physicians who can provide their expertise regarding the likelihood that an injury is the result of abuse.

The REACH program was started fifteen years ago, a concept conceived by Dr. Lenane and two other pediatricians. "Child Protective Service caseworkers were sending abused children to the hospital's Emergency Department," she says. "We three pediatricians knew these children would need comprehensive evaluations. We proposed to leadership that we begin a once-a-month clinic for these children." Now a full-time clinic operating off-campus at the Bivona Child Advocacy Center in downtown Rochester, the REACH program provides more than six hundred evaluations a year, including referrals from regional hospitals, as well as health and human service providers.

Supervisor Bob Barnes of Monroe County's CPS knows Dr. Lenane well; they have been working together for twenty-five years. "Ann is passionate about her work. She sees how abuse affects not just the victims, but their families. Part of her work is focused on finding ways to prevent it." Barnes notes that when CPS caseworkers confront cases involving difficult medical issues—such as brittle bone diseases, bleeding disorders, or Munchausen by Proxy—Dr. Lenane can turn to expert colleagues who are part of her network, both at the University of Rochester and across the nation. Her knowledge of the field, he says, has helped educate those working in the legal system and its courts of law, where she frequently appears as an expert witness.

As professor of pediatrics, clinician, and administrator, Dr. Lenane also teaches medical students, residents, and fellows, sharing what she has learned about child abuse during her quarter of a century working in the field. Still more hours are designated to collaborating with colleagues around the country on the best ways to confront the rising national tide of child abuse.

How does a woman, herself a mother, manage in this intense emotional hothouse? "It helps to be an optimist," says Dr. Lenane. "It *is* a challenging field. Our best moments come when we see a success, when years later we meet a child whom we've helped who now is living a better life. We review our failures, looking for ways to improve that might save others."

For Ann Lenane, growing up in Rochester in the 1970s was a sunny time. She found pleasure in being "big sister" to her siblings while her mother worked and babysitting for lively neighborhood children. As Ann's college years approached, she had narrowed her career focus to teaching or nursing. A computer program (then a relative rarity) in her high school guidance office recommended the University of Dayton, which offered qualified students in the education program the opportunity to begin student teaching as a sophomore. A well-regarded Catholic college, Dayton also offered a generous financial package, important for the young woman who would be the first in her family to attend college.

Sometime during that pre-college summer, Ann changed her mind about her choice of major. She had read an article by a pediatric surgeon who described his satisfaction in using his skill to mend children; she was impressed. "I wrote a letter to the college asking to change my major from education to biology," she says. "I was encouraged by my parents, who taught us that we could do anything we put our minds to."

Dayton, a midsize university, was just right for Ann. Small classes, especially in biology, gave her an opportunity to work with supportive professors. Her first philosophy class focused on medical ethics and the topic reinforced her new focus. An unexpected roadblock loomed when her father suddenly lost his job, but her family found a way to allow her to complete her four years and graduate *magna cum laude*.

In 1978, Ann entered medical school at State University of New York Upstate Medical University in Syracuse. As a first-year medical student, Ann was uncomfortable with the didactic curriculum, wondering if she had made the right choice when she decided to become a physician. Anatomy was especially difficult, bringing on twenty-four-hour headaches that lasted for a month. "I told the dean my doubts about whether medicine was the right choice for me. He sent me to see Dr. John Wolf, a sympathetic neurologist on the faculty. He helped by taking me, a new medical student, into his clinic once a week to observe. Working with him was so inspiring that I knew I had made the right choice." Ann became so intrigued that she took a six-week elective in neurology before beginning her clinical rotations.

During those rotations, Ann found the most satisfaction in caring for children; she decided to become a pediatrician. She also discovered a passion for working in the emergency room. "In the ED, you have to figure things out with only a minimal amount of information available," she says. "The women and men who work there are people who can handle the stress of dealing fast and effectively with critically ill or injured patients."

In 1982, Ann received her medical degree—and she began her internship at a time when interns were sometimes required to work thirty-six hours at a stretch. "Working at night alone in the Pediatric ED was the most terrifying," Ann says, "when the only backup help was the resident far away up on the fourth floor." She learned what was needed to survive: "Don't whine—and drink lots of coffee."

"At that time, the pediatrics program at Syracuse was rather like Camelot, a special window of time that brought together faculty who would become leaders in the field," she says. The elite group had been brought together by Frank A. Oski, MD, who later would chair the Department of Pediatrics at Johns Hopkins University; he also founded the journal *Contemporary Pediatrics*. As a professor, Dr. Oski was both tough and intimidating, Dr. Lenane recalls. "He was looking for residents with backbone," she says. She was one of them.

In contrast to Dr. Oski, her advisor, Walter W. Tunnessen, Jr., MD, was kind, gentle, and a brilliant clinician. (Dr. Tunnessen, who ran the ambulatory pediatrics program, would eventually win every major medical teaching award at State University of New York Upstate Medical University in Syracuse, University of Pennsylvania's Children's Hospital, and Johns Hopkins University.) "I learned so much about the art as well as the science of medicine as I watched him work with children and their families," she says.

During the third year of her residency at SUNY Upstate Medical University, Ann married fellow resident William (Bill) Varade, now a pediatric nephrologist in the Department of Pediatrics. She began thinking about the future, children, and family and how they might fit into a career. The prevailing wisdom of the time was that a good fit was impossible. However, pediatric emergency medicine seemed to offer some flexibility in work scheduling, making it possible to combine career and family.

Ann had learned both at home and at college the importance of "giving back" to a needy world. With her residency almost completed, the time seemed right to look for outreach work before she and Bill began their fellowship years. Bill and Ann had been able to secure fellowships at the Children's Hospital of Cincinnati; Bill in pediatric nephrology and Ann in ambulatory and emergency pediatrics, both programs that allowed them to defer their fellowships for a year. The young doctors had found an overseas healthcare center in American Samoa that needed not just one but two pediatricians. The center fit their bill perfectly: almost half of the island residents were children and most needed medical care.

When their term in Samoa ended, Ann and Bill returned to Cincinnati to begin their fellowships. During their fellowships, a life-changing event occurred—the birth of their first child (a boy named William Stephen III, after his father and recently deceased grandfather). While Bill was completing the third year of his nephrology fellowship, Ann took a job with an independent pediatric practitioner. She worked three days a week in the practice, also taking emergency room shifts at the Children's Hospital. This schedule enabled her to compare working in a practice with working in an academic emergency department before deciding what the next step in her career would be. She chose the emergency department.

By 1989, Ann and Bill needed to find faculty positions in a community where they could work and raise the son who had been born during their fellowship years, as well as their second child, soon to be born. They wanted a medium-size city with an excellent pediatric department—and the UR Medical Center at that time needed another pediatric nephrologist. Bill was hired, and Ann began work as an emergency pediatrician. She was encouraged to pursue a master's in Public Health, and this meant starting her first class when her baby daughter was two weeks old. Six weeks later, when she returned to full-time work in addition to taking a graduate class and having a family, she was overwhelmed. "I was exhausted, ready to lose my mind," she says of those stressful days.

Ann uses that difficult moment as a teaching example when she mentors young faculty. "Women of my day often had too high expectations," she says. "We really thought we could do it all. That often leads to bad decision-making." Ann was given sound and supportive advice from Peter Szilagyi, MD, then director of the fellowship program. He saw that Ann would only be satisfied when working at the top of her game. "Just now you're carrying the weight of the world on your shoulders. You could work part-time." Her request was supported by Lance Rodewald, MD, then head of pediatric emergency medicine. Today, pointing out the danger of professional burnout and teaching ways to prevent it has become an important part of Dr. Lenane's educational mission.

Ann's first appointment at the URMC was as a clinical instructor in emergency medicine. Over the next twenty-five years, she advanced up the ladder in both emergency medicine and pediatrics as senior instructor, assistant professor, associate professor of pediatrics, and, in 2018, full professor of pediatrics. Along the way, she has forged partnerships with faculty and staff at Strong Memorial and Golisano Children's Hospital, other regional hospitals, and within the community.

Over the years Dr. Lenane's relationships within her specialty have also strengthened. She has been active on many national and state committees including the Violence Prevention Committee of the New York State Chapter of the American Academy of Pediatrics; the Child Abuse Mentorship Program in New York State; the Best Practices Committee of the New York Chapter of the American Professional Society on Child Abuse; and the Mental Health Committee of the Ray Helfer Society.

Dr. Elizabeth Murray, a REACH physician and one of Dr. Lenane's mentees, says her own career decision to work with abused children was shaped when she was a medical student at the University of New England College of Osteopathic Medicine. "Ann's career course matches my own, and I've been able to learn from her years of experience, both as a clinician and as a teacher. She is always there when I face a difficult problem, never telling me what to do, but helping me reach my own solution. My speed dial consists of my husband, my parents, and Ann."

Dr. Lenane says she is proud of the fact that she has been able to navigate her career in her own way. At the same time, she has succeeded in making a difference in a difficult field—all while working part-time. With children now grown (William III, a law student at St. John's University, and Marissa

Lenane Varade, pursuing a master's degree in marine science at Northeastern University), this avid equestrian relishes spending free time on horseback, as well as jogging, biking, and traveling with her husband.

Ann Lenane's advice for young people entering the field matches her own career style. "Think hard about what you want your life to be like, including the role of family and friends. In choosing a career, talk with people in your chosen field and learn what the expectations will be. Along the way, bend—but not too much. The destination is important, but so is the journey."

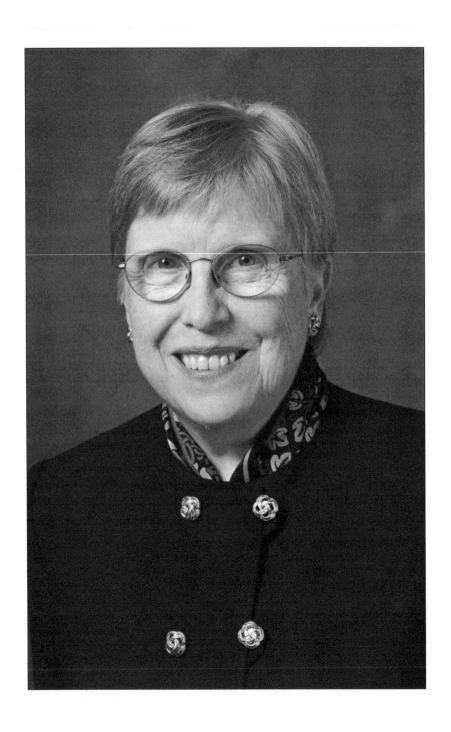

Chapter Twenty-Two

ELIZABETH R. McANARNEY, MD

"It's all about the children. It's always about the children." Those words best identify the woman who for years has been a leader in the charge to create our local hallmark of children's healthcare in upstate New York, The Golisano Children's Hospital at Strong of the University of Rochester.

In 2018, Dr. Elizabeth McAnarney was given the rare honor of being the first woman to be named a Distinguished University Professor, becoming only the thirteenth recipient of the honor in the university's history. In announcing the acknowledgement, then University of Rochester President Joel Seligman said, "Dr. McAnarney's contributions to the community and to pediatric health at large cannot be overstated. She has given all of herself to Rochester, and to our children, for the past fifty years."

Joie de vivre, devotion to her profession, and indefatigable energy all mark Dr. McAnarney's half century of dedication to pediatrics. She has been clinician, researcher, teacher, mentor, fundraiser, and community advocate for all things related to children's health, rising from a young research fellow in the late 1960s to chair of the Department of Pediatrics.

Over the years, Dr. McAnarney led changes in the breadth and scope of the Department of Pediatrics. With colleagues, she broadcast a new message: that adolescents, a forgotten group, needed health providers with special expertise who can guide teenagers through this challenging time. Soon, the University of Rochester's adolescent medicine program became a national model of care, training, and research, with young pediatricians from across the country coming to Rochester. "Nationally, Lissa is among the most influential individuals in adolescent medicine. That field would not be what it is today without her influence and advocacy," says Mark Taubman, MD, CEO of the University of Rochester Medical Center and dean of the School of Medicine and Dentistry.

Dr. McAnarney's election in 2000 to the Institute of Medicine (now the National Academy of Medicine) of the National Academy of Sciences recognizes the importance of her work. The list of her partnerships and achievements reaches beyond her own specialty and deep into our nation's community of medical colleagues. In 2013, Dr. McAnarney was awarded the American Pediatric Society's John Howland Medal, the highest lifetime achievement award in pediatrics.

She has presided over three major professional organizations: the American Pediatric Society; the Association of Medical School Pediatric Department Chairs (the first woman elected to lead the group); and the Society for Adolescent Medicine. She has been an advisor to the Robert Wood Johnson Foundation, the Food and Drug Administration, and has served on several National Institutes of Health special study groups.

During her years as chair of the Department of Pediatrics, from 1993 to 2006, Dr. McAnarney led upstate New York's premier pediatric program, then a multimillion-dollar-a-year enterprise that in 1998 ranked thirteenth among pediatric departments in NIH funding. Author or co-author of nearly 150 papers and chapters, she is chief editor of the *Textbook of Adolescent Medicine*.

Still hard at work on the children's health issues, Elizabeth McAnarney has the perspective to see how her life's work has benefitted generations of children and their families.

"Lissa" McAnarney grew up in Watkins Glen, NY, a picturesque lakeside community of 2,500 residents. "Our mother and father were highly supportive of the educations of their three daughters. We had aunts who were teachers on both sides of our family and the professions of education and nursing were popular options for women."

Early on, Lissa learned how hard work and creativity resulted in rewards. Her first business endeavor occurred at age seven, when her father "hired" her to shine his shoes for a stipend. A businessman, he discussed a business plan, developed an income and expense sheet, and explained that she must pay for her own supplies. Lissa had her own bank account and deposited income each month, "richly supplemented by our mother's occasional contributions."

Soon, Lissa supplemented her college fund by seeking out—and often winning—popular contests sponsored by product manufacturers, including a prize-winning essay, "The Importance of the Concord Grape in Upstate New York's Economy." (She was prescient in choosing that subject, she realizes, considering the Finger Lakes' important role in today's wine world.)

It was Vassar College that channeled Lissa's energy and opened the doors to a life of research into the fluidly changing lives of children and adolescents. The college during the late 1950s and 1960s was home to an innovative laboratory nursery school where Vassar students observed youngsters playing and interacting under the watchful eyes of specially trained educators. Dr. McAnarney says, "In retrospect, I learned more at Vassar firsthand about child development than I did at any other time during my education. Much was expected of each student. My term paper on 'parallel play' was more like a master's thesis."

"Training at a laboratory nursery school was seminal for me," says Dr. McAnarney. As an undergraduate, standing at the nursery school door, carefully observing and recording the children's interactions, Lissa McAnarney surely was unaware of the distinguished career that lay ahead.

Even though few women were accepted at medical schools during the mid-sixties, McAnarney refused to be discouraged. After graduating from Vassar in 1962, she began her medical training at State University of New York Upstate Medical University in Syracuse. In her class of 1966, there were five women and ninety-five men. Lissa remembers her days as a medical student as packed with hard work. "You either performed at a consistently high level or you were openly chastised," she says. As a resident, the work was grueling: thirty-six hours on and twelve hours off.

It was as a first-year student that she met a professor who would become a significant mentor, Julius B. Richmond, MD, then chair of pediatrics and dean of the medical school in Syracuse. Dr. Richmond at that time was introducing elements of psychiatry into the practice of pediatrics. His message would be transformative. Inspired by the 1954 Supreme Court case Brown vs. Board of Education, Richmond's cognitive research documented how poverty—including malnutrition—threatened the psychosocial development of children. (In later years, Dr. Richmond would help change American social policy, as co-founder of Project Head Start and as US surgeon general during Jimmy Carter's term as president from 1976 to 1980.)

Syracuse was such a perfect fit for McAnarney that, after graduating from medical school with honors in 1966, she would stay for her pediatric residency. In 1967, Dr. Richmond arranged for Lissa to meet Dr. Robert J. Haggerty, chair of pediatrics at the University of Rochester, who had funds for an important new fellowship in behavioral pediatrics. The interview was momentous: The University of Rochester Medical Center would become the focus of Dr. McAnarney's life for at least the next fifty years.

In Rochester, Lissa's fellowship work in behavioral pediatrics and adolescent medicine took a giant step forward when Dr. Haggerty introduced her to her next mentor, Stanford B. Friedman, MD. Friedman at the time was developing an innovative curriculum in behavioral pediatrics and adolescent medicine.

Dr. Friedman had faith in even the uninitiated. Lissa arrived in Rochester to begin her fellowship in behavioral pediatrics and adolescent medicine on July 1, 1968, having stayed up until midnight the night before as the supervising resident in Syracuse. Dr. Friedman's words of greeting were, "There's a patient waiting on B-4 for you to complete a consultation." As Lissa recalls, "I thought, I don't even know where B-4 is. I don't know anything about behavioral pediatrics, and I need to put my bag down and find a place to sit."

Dr. Friedman was, she says, one of the most brilliant fellowship directors she has ever met. "He pushed us way beyond what we imagined we could do. Stan became a mentor and friend for me, as he was for many." In 1972, Dr. McAnarney followed Dr. Friedman as director of the adolescent medicine program, a post she held for twenty-two years. She was succeeded by Richard E. Kreipe, MD, one of her former fellows, who held the post for twelve years.

Beginning in the early 1960s, Dr. Haggerty was working to connect trainees with Rochester's "inner city," where many families lived in poverty. As part of Dr. Haggerty's program, Lissa became involved with an innovative community program targeting pregnant teenagers at high medical risk. The Rochester Adolescent Maternity Program (RAMP) provided comprehensive obstetrical and psychosocial care for young mothers at Strong Memorial Hospital and linked them, their babies, and their families with other social services within the community. RAMP became the site of Dr. McAnarney's subsequent years of research, work that dispelled the myth that the high-risk mother-infant dyad was at greater risk of morbidity and mortality than adults based solely on maternal age.

In 1993, Dr. Elizabeth McAnarney became the sixth chair of the Department of Pediatrics and Pediatrician-in-Chief at the University of Rochester. (She had served for the past three years as acting and associate chair consecutively.) As the twenty-first century approached, she saw her role clearly: Help the department transition to the future.

Dr. McAnarney brought to the department a simple, no-nonsense philosophy: children are our first priority; excellence is expected from everyone; investments will be made in focused programs of excellence; and accountability to children, parents, and the community (including the university) is expected of everyone. The new chair understood the budget's importance, especially at a time when managed care contracts were limiting clinical services and when federal funding for research and training grants was severely restricted.

"Today a chair's job is managing a business, a highly regulated business that is shaped by external forces," she told an interviewer. This was not the role she had prepared for during her early years in Rochester, and earlier at Syracuse and Vassar. Undaunted, she was ready for the challenge—and a challenge it was. During the preceding decade, four key faculty had left to become chairs at other institutions. She began her tenure by recruiting heavily; over the next years she would hire eight new division chiefs, leaders in pediatric programs in general academic pediatrics, adolescent medicine, cardiology, pulmonology, infectious diseases, gastroenterology, hematology-oncology, and neonatology.

A new Children's Heart Center was established, and a research initiative in cardiomyopathy reflected the interest of the new chief from Boston Children's Hospital. A new suite for young patients and their families honored longtime chief of pediatric cardiology Dr. James Manning. A consolidated Rochester-Buffalo-Syracuse congenital heart center was developed, with Strong Memorial's cardiovascular surgeon Dr. George Alfieris performing surgery in Rochester on children from all three cities. Faculty were recruited for most divisions, and Dr. McAnarney nourished and expanded partnerships between pediatrics faculty and surgeons.

Strong Memorial's new Neonatal Intensive Care Unit, developed under the supervision of chief of neonatology Dale L. Phelps, MD, opened in 1993. As the NICU responded to a growing need—more beds for critically ill newborns—so, in 1996, did the hospital's new ambulatory care facility.

"We're in the middle of a biomedical explosion," said Dr. McAnarney in 1998. "Yet all the wonderful discoveries won't mean a thing unless we take these advances directly to our children." In the midst of all this activity, one goal—long envisioned by every chair since the medical school's founding in 1926—remained unfulfilled: a children's hospital associated with the University of Rochester. All the chairs knew its potential value—both moral and financial. The problem over all those years: How can we build a fiscally sound base for a multimillion-dollar operation?

President Joel Seligman made funding the new hospital a priority of the university's historic capital campaign (2011–16). The creation of the current Golisano Children's Hospital was accelerated by an original $14 million and subsequent $20 million donated by B. Thomas Golisano, founder of the Paychex corporation. In addition to Dr. McAnarney, other catalysts helping bring the hospital project to fruition were the university's Board of Trustees, president of the university, medical and hospital leadership, and volunteer fundraisers.

Not all leaders are alike. Jonathan Klein, MD, spent eighteen years in Rochester, working in the Department of Pediatrics, before leaving for an executive post at the American Academy of Pediatrics. Dr. Klein sees what makes this leader different. "Lissa has always had the ability to see all the people on her team as individuals, at the same time that she's somehow equally focused on her profession and the institution. She cares about her students, her residents, and interns. She knows their names, their children's names, their pets. She's helped in this by her secretary of forty-three years, Carole M. Berger. A wonderfully complementary team, they make things run smoothly." (Or as smoothly as they can in a hospital, where crises inevitably occur every day.)

Dr. Richard E. Kreipe, the Elizabeth R. McAnarney Professor of Pediatrics, adds: "I've seen Lissa stand toe-to-toe with academic leaders at the highest level of authority, always committed to what is right for children and families. She advocates for others, not for herself."

At a time when healthcare may seem institutionalized, the insights that Elizabeth McAnarney has brought to pediatrics are more important than ever. Redefining "the big picture," the vision required to respond to changing times and changing needs, is vitally important. But that goal is easier to reach when those working to achieve it are acknowledged and valued.

As for Elizabeth McAnarney's own goal, that continues to be crystal clear: "It's about the children. It's always about the children."

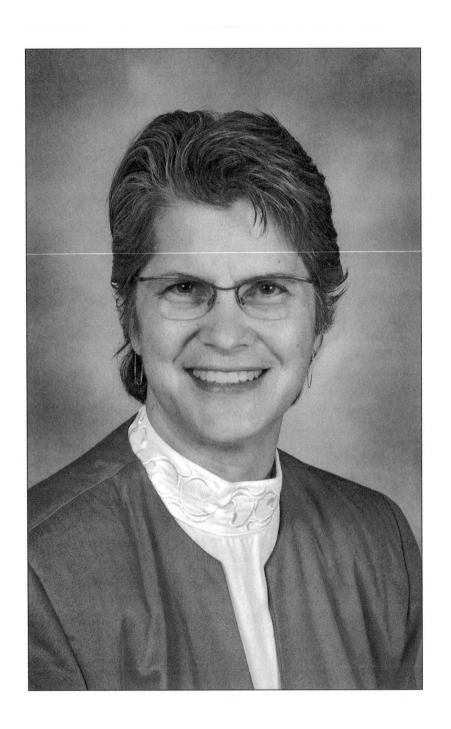

Chapter Twenty-Three

DALE L. PHELPS, MD

Dr. Dale Phelps is nationally known for her research mission: finding and promoting ways to prevent and treat Retinopathy of Prematurity (ROP), which affects the eyesight of many babies born earlier than thirty-four weeks gestation. ROP is a condition in which normal growth of the retinal blood vessels has been disrupted by exposure to higher oxygen levels than they would have experienced in the uterus. These infants are at high risk for visual impairment or blindness from the bleeding and scarring that occurs in the eyes as the retina attempts to control that abnormal vessel growth.

At the University of Rochester in the 1980s, Dr. Phelps continued the laboratory research on ROP she began at the University of California, Los Angeles. She joined the national team of ophthalmologists, led by Earl Palmer, MD, designing the first multicenter clinical trial of cryotherapy to treat this sight-robbing disease and applying the new classification system of ROP developed in anticipation of the trial. Together with the Department of Ophthalmology, Neonatology at the UR was one of the participating centers that found cryotherapy was so effective for moderately severe ROP that the controlled trial was stopped early to speed its implementation as accepted treatment. Based on the trial, cryotherapy therapy (later replaced by laser treatment) became the standard of care for treating severe ROP, and all preterm infants were carefully examined to detect the disease early, a major change in practice. At the time, UR chief of neonatology Donald Shapiro said, "Dr. Phelps's research is a remarkable example of how quickly science can move from research to practice."

Dr. Phelps continued her pioneering studies in the laboratory, studying the effects of vitamin E on oxygen-induced retinopathy first in an animal model, followed by a randomized controlled trial for infants, both funded by the National Eye Institute (NEI), a division of the NIH. The vitamin E studies did not show effectiveness for preventing ROP, a fact that was important to know. Her later research on the effectiveness of oxygen-limiting protocols led in 1994 to the important STOP-ROP clinical trial, in which supplemental oxygen was carefully administered at one of two different levels to premature babies who had already developed ROP. STOP-ROP was funded by both the NIH/NEI and the Eunice Kennedy Shriver National Institute of Child Health and Human Development (NICHD) Neonatal Research Network.

Thousands of premature infants have benefitted from the research done by Dr. Phelps in collaboration with the dedicated ophthalmologists she has worked with. She is quick to point out that only by working together with others who share a common vision is such progress possible. In 2010 Dr. Phelps received the Landmark Award from the American Academy of Pediatrics's Perinatal Section for Lifetime Contributions to the understanding and treatment of ROP.

Dale greatly admired her father, an anesthesiologist. She knew early on that like her father, she too wanted to be an Eagle Scout and to help people as a doctor. She vividly remembers the day when she asked her father, "Can a nurse set a broken arm?" When her father said "No," she responded, "Well, then I'll have to be a doctor!" and walked away. (Fortunately, she adds, that turned out better than the flat refusal of the Boy Scouts of America to accept girls into their program.)

At Pomona College in Claremont, California, Dale completed her pre-med courses in three years and applied to several medical schools, but to none of those who stated they did not accept women. Interviews were generally cordial and encouraging, but one interviewer asked, "What's your hurry, little girl?" Her response: "Why should my father pay for another year of college when I've completed my entrance requirements?" In 1969, she was accepted at Northwestern University's Feinberg School of Medicine in Chicago.

Dale so enjoyed medical school and her many differing clinical rotations that "Not until the day before Match Day selection deadline did I realize I really wanted to be a pediatrician. I wanted to be there at the beginning, a place where I could help and teach and learn." She completed her pediatric internships and residency at Children's Memorial Hospital in Chicago in 1971.

Summer preceptorships were invaluable for preparing Dale for the career that would follow, one in anesthesiology during medical school at Harbor General Hospital in Torrance, California; a second in neonatology with John Boehm, MD, at Evanston Hospital in Evanston, Illinois, just prior to her internship; and a third in perinatal medicine at the UR School of Medicine and Dentistry between residency and fellowship in 1971 where she studied with Mortimer Rosen, MD, and first met UR's lactation specialist Ruth Lawrence, MD.

While at Pomona College, Dale met Charles (Chuck) Phelps. Their value systems and vision of marriage and life meshed perfectly, she says. "Chuck's ability to work successfully with people was influenced by his high school experience of spending summers as a camp counselor at the Easter Seal Handicamps. Chuck helped campers deal with all kinds of obstacles, for example the blind boy in archery class who learned to hit the target by aiming at the ringing bell behind it." Chuck also moved to Chicago, beginning graduate studies at the University of Chicago. He and Dale were married two years later.

Relocating after Dale's residency and Chuck's PhD completion was the first of several dual career challenges the couple has faced. When Chuck decided to accept his first PhD post with the Rand Corporation in California, Dale found that her supervisors from summer preceptor experiences were invaluable as references. They helped her secure a last-minute fellowship in neonatology at a site near where Chuck was working.

For Dale, three years of a neonatology fellowship within the UCLA Hospital systems followed at St. Mary Medical Center, Long Beach, California; and at Harbor-UCLA Medical Center, Torrence, California. There she experienced her first exposure to and participation in laboratory research with William Oh, MD. Her passion to learn about what became known as Retinopathy of Prematurity was sparked there while attending a follow-up clinic for neonatal graduates when a one-year-old boy was brought in "because his eyes dance." Dr. Phelps arranged an appointment with an ophthalmologist who diagnosed Retrolental Fibroplasia (RLF) and explained that the boy was blind. Until then, Dale had had no clinical encounter with this disorder in her rotations and only minimal discussion of why oxygen use had to be strictly limited to only what the baby needs to avoid hypoxia.

That encounter occurred within days of her reading a newly published report that the incidence of RLF/ROP was increasing as ever-greater numbers of premature infants were surviving. Dale also learned that two scientific presentations on the subject were scheduled that very month at the Pediatric Academic Society meetings, one describing the relationship of oxygen use and preterm birth and one a clinical study reporting the use of vitamin E in premature infants to prevent ROP.

As Dale began her first faculty appointment at the UCLA Medical Center at Los Angeles, she proposed and secured an NIH grant from the National Eye Institute to study vitamin E in an animal model of ROP. These studies led to a small randomized trial to determine if using vitamin E to prevent ROP in premature infants would be safe and effective. As trial results were reported, Dr. William Silverman, "one of the most important historians on Neonatal Intensive Care—and particularly RLF/ROP," reached out to Dale. He would become a great friend and mentor.

In what Dale calls "the next great adventure," a UCLA colleague alerted her to an upcoming meeting of ophthalmologists in Chicago where a multicenter trial of a surgical treatment for early ROP would be discussed. She hopped on a plane and soon met the man who would become a new research colleague. Earl Palmer, MD, a pediatric ophthalmologist at the Oregon Health and Sciences University, was planning a grant proposal to the NEI to conduct a multicenter clinical trial to determine if cryotherapy as treatment for ROP would be effective and safe. To protect infants from what might not be an effective surgery or might have late complications, only one eye would be treated. After Dr. Palmer's presentation at the meeting, Dale introduced herself and asked, "Do you have a neonatologist working with your group? If not, you want me on your planning committee. Dr. Palmer, boarded in both ophthalmology and pediatrics, smiled in his usual gracious manner and invited me to the next Planning Committee meeting," Dale recalls. As a member of Palmer's team, Dr. Phelps helped develop and run the very successful trial.

As Dr. Phelps's career advanced, her friend "Bill" Silverman continued to be a cherished, outspoken critic. "He was a critical scientific thinker whose landmark work on Retrolental Fibroplasia was coupled with unflinching advocacy for safety, for scientific rigor in clinical trials, and for long-term follow-up," she says. "He was most gracious in sharing his time, encouragement, networking, and integrity."

At UCLA, as Dale progressed to associate professor of medicine, the Phelps family grew to include a son and a daughter. "Together the family discussed and found ways to reach out for the assistance we needed to help raise these wonderful kids, while both of us were working full-time and I was often 'on call' at night. Flexibility and reaching out to seek solutions really work!" she says.

After ten years spent in California in their first positions, it was time to consider the next step. Since Chuck had several tempting offers they decided to optimize the choice based on its value for him, its potential for Dale, and on the quality of schooling for their children, Darin and Teresa, now eight and ten years of age. Chuck was eager to move into the academic challenges of a major university where he could best use his skills. "I was certain that Rochester would need another neonatologist," Dale says, "because neonatology was a rapidly expanding specialty in those days—and Rochester's schools and the community itself looked great."

This indeed was a seminal time for UR Neonatology, led by researchers Dr. Robert Notter, Dr. Donald Shapiro, and Dr. Jacob Finkelstein, who, as noted earlier, had pioneered the use of surfactant refined from calves' lungs to treat babies born with immature lungs. However, at that time, the neonatology division had a full complement of clinicians. As Dale described her research goals and skills, Dr. Shapiro suggested this might be a good time academically for her to have a research year. Following his advice, Dale began a research fellowship with Dr. Victor Laites in toxicology.

The change proved to be extremely timely (and successful), allowing Dale to contribute significantly to the developing national ROP studies and to secure research funding. The first step was to develop an ROP classification of prognostic value that could be used everywhere consistently. The protocol required that all babies born prematurely in the hospital have their eyes examined by an ophthalmologist before being released to their home; informed parental consent was required; and the findings were recorded in very specific ways that had been worked out collaboratively.

This was a serious change in practice for most participating centers, since previously no discharge exams were being done. The new rule resulted in scheduling complications for ophthalmologists and NICU pediatricians, nurses, and staff. "The study proved the usefulness of the International Classification of ROP and the timing of ROP progression and was critical to conducting the controlled trial of treatment," says Dr. Phelps. "It required review by the Institutional Review Board and approval, a lot of diplomacy, conferences, teaching, and informed consent—just for starters! Never underestimate the time it takes, or the value of explaining the background—the 'why'—to staff, families, and professionals involved. I even learned how to make a video explaining the disease and the research for staff and families."

During this valuable year, Dr. Phelps was able to attend the Department of Pediatrics's clinical and research meetings, which enabled her to get to know the faculty and to learn how the division functioned. Dr. William Maniscalco's research on the effects of oxygen and ventilation on immature lungs complemented her own investigations, and the ongoing discussion of oxygen toxicity was ever present. A very special moment for her was being able to observe the effects of the first surfactant administered to human infants. "The effect was remarkable," she says, and knowledge of what could be done to help these infants was exploding.

Dr. Shapiro added Dr. Phelps to the Department of Pediatrics faculty after that year, and she was able to continue her funded research with her ROP colleagues. After the untimely death of Dr. Shapiro in 1989, she was appointed division chief in neonatology, serving until 2000 when Dr. Maniscalco was appointed to that role. Dr. Phelps successfully competed for the division to join the Eunice Kennedy Shriver NICHD Neonatal Research Network and she remained as a full-time faculty member until she and Chuck retired in 2008.

Even after Dr. Phelps formally "retired" from her full-time position at the university, she has continued her academic work on ROP. She was the principal investigator on a twenty-two center, randomized trial testing an earlier hypothesis based on smaller studies studying the promising efficacy of inositol, a natural sugar, to prevent ROP. Unfortunately it was determined that the inositol did not improve ROP but actually increased other adverse effects. Since other centers were using inositol in the treatment of ROP off-label, it was critical that professional colleagues treating infants who have ROP knew of the important findings from Dr. Phelps's and colleagues' research.

Thus, there are at least two lessons in Dr. Phelps's post-retirement work. The first is that one does not have to stop thinking after one retires! Second, it is imperative that colleagues are made aware of the results of well-designed studies that yield data that do not support the original hypothesis (in this instance that inositol might help improve ROP), particularly when patients might suffer unexpected adverse effects of the treatment not previously identified fully.

Although Dale and Chuck Phelps now live in California, daughter Teresa Phelps Schoell has forged a career in Rochester as head of the Child Life Program at Rochester General Hospital. Son Darin, after graduating from UR, had a career in musical theater in Manhattan and now directs the program in computer IT development at the New York University's Law School.

Over the years, Dale Phelps has negotiated the path linking professional achievement and a satisfying family life. She has this advice for young people beginning their careers in medicine:

- Don't be afraid to ask questions and to ask for help.
- Network. Listen to others and offer back thoughts and insights as you have them.
- It's important to talk with colleagues. Learn how they have met challenges.
- Test your scientific ideas by sharing them with colleagues, to anyone who will listen, and best of all, to those who will ask you really tough questions.
- Some of my best advice came from people outside my field.
- Always remember to respect confidences, and to recognize and thank those who have shared their wisdom.

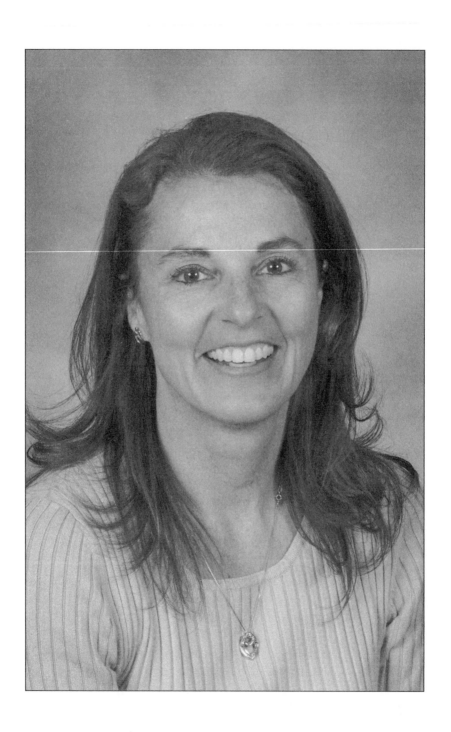

Chapter Twenty-Four

KAREN S. POWERS, MD

Dr. Karen Power's world is the rapidly changing, potentially life-or-death environment of a pediatric intensive care unit, the PICU. She shares that world, night and day, with a dedicated group of critical care doctors and nurses who consider themselves a family. "We're like brothers and sisters," Powers says. "We're always there to support each other, as we work together to bring our critically ill or injured patients back to health."

As a girl growing up in Charleston, South Carolina, Karen didn't expect to become a doctor. She loved animals and thought she might want to become a veterinarian. In high school and during her first two years of college (Furman University in Greenville, South Carolina), biology was her favorite subject. When her father died during her sophomore year at Furman, Karen moved back home and that autumn transferred to the College of Charleston. Fortunately, her new academic home had a strong biology program that supported her growing interest. Karen graduated in 1978 with a bachelor's degree in science.

That degree led her immediately to a job in a research laboratory in neurochemistry at the Medical University of South Carolina (MUSC) where she worked with neuroscientists who were investigating the effects of spinal trauma on rats. In addition to running chemical assays, Karen's job was to surgically expose the rats' spinal cords and systematically incur blunt trauma to the spinal cord. "I discovered I really liked hands-on technical work—and I was good at it," she says.

As a medical student at MUSC in Charleston, Karen's interest in surgery continued. But when her pediatric rotation began, her focus suddenly shifted.

"Kids are so resilient, so upbeat. Unlike adults, who often have confounding problems, children have 'pure disease.' They're generally healthy except for the one thing that's wrong with them. When that problem is resolved, it often fades like a glitch on their life's radar."

Karen received her medical degree in 1984 and continued on at the university for her pediatric residency. She knew by then that her medical focus would be on the sickest children, spending as much time as possible in the hospital's converted four-bed intensive care unit. The medical center completed a new children's tower the same year Karen completed her residency training and she became a resident fellow in the Divisions of Pediatric Cardiology and Critical Care, working for one year in the newly opened PICU dedicated to children with medical problems, including illness, trauma, and post-surgical care.

The medical director of the PICU at Charleston was Dr. Frederick Techlenburg, who would become a mentor for Dr. Powers. "Fred had energy, passion, and dedication that was unequalled. He gave me independence, but I always knew he was there to help if I needed it," she says, working in the newly opened twelve-bed PICU. For the next year, Dr. Powers would train with "Dr. Fred," working all day in the PICU, plus on call every other night and weekend. "I learned so much," she says, "about intubation, central venous access, and treating abnormal heart rhythms."

Following the recruitment of her husband Jim as chief of neuropathology at Columbia University, she moved to White Plains, New York, and completed her critical care fellowship at the Albert Einstein College of Medicine, training in PICUs at Montefiore Medical Center and Jacobi Hospital. Her research focused on the pharmacokinetics of new sedative-type medications. Her co-fellow there was Dr. Edward Conway, who later became chair of pediatrics at Beth Israel Hospital. "Together we were a force to be reckoned with," says Powers with a smile. "For two years, we covered two ICUs at two different hospitals, traveling back and forth between them every day."

Critical care as a subspecialty was then in its infancy. "I fell in love with critical care," Dr. Powers says of the work that would become her career focus.

"I liked the action, the acuity, the technology, the challenge. Things happen fast in the ICU. There's always something new to learn. It suited my personality." During the late 1980s, change was coming at medical training programs across the country. The realization was growing that doctors, nurses, anesthesiologists, and technicians with special training were needed to support not only people with medical problems, but also the growing numbers of surgical patients who required mechanical ventilatory support as they transitioned from the operating room.

In 1990, Dr. Powers was offered a position as an attending physician at Schneider Children's Hospital of Long Island Jewish Medical Center. "These two years at Long Island were very exciting," she says, "I especially liked working with the cardiac patients, where we would see acute changes happen fast. Often patients would transition from being very ill to returning home in four days."

The late 1980s were challenging years for hospitals, especially in New York City, Karen recalls. "The HIV epidemic was at its peak," she says, "and it was difficult to recruit doctors, nurses, and researchers to big cities." Real fear gripped the city; so much was unknown about this new plague. When the stock market crashed, the combined effect on hospitals was devastating. In 1992, Columbia Medical Center was losing a million dollars a week and operating with skeleton crews.

On the domestic scene, Karen's commute from White Plains into the city was challenging, especially for a PICU doctor. (To handle emergency calls, she travelled with one of the new, bulky portable phones, so large that it filled her car's passenger seat.) "We were both dissatisfied," she recalls. For the Powers family, it was time to move on.

However, when Jim Powers returned from an interview at the University of Rochester with the news that he really liked Rochester "and they really, really want you, too," Karen's Southern roots manifested. As she thought of sunny beaches and the horses she loved to ride, she demurred. "Have you forgotten where South is?" she asked. "I'll look [at Rochester]," she told him, "but I won't like it . . ." In fact, she *did* like it, and she also liked Dr. Robert Hoekelman, then chair of pediatrics, and the pediatric critical care team that Dr. Jeffery Rubenstein was assembling. With their arrival in 1992, the university acquired both a chief of neuropathology *and* a pediatric critical care specialist.

For the next several years, Dr. Powers, Dr. Jeffrey Rubenstein, and others worked to strengthen and grow the PICU at Strong Memorial Hospital, which has expanded from the original eight-bed unit to twenty-two beds, and soon it will expand to twenty-six. Originally the PICU served only children with medical problems. A major change came in the late 1990s when Strong Memorial became the principal pediatric cardiac surgical center for the upstate hospital consortium for Rochester, Buffalo, and Syracuse. The expanding pediatric surgical programs, and especially the cardiothoracic program, demanded a need for more ICU beds. "The pediatric surgeons recognized our expertise in helping support these patients and, with the blessings of the relevant department chairs, our PICU program expanded," Powers explains. Thirteen pediatric intensivists now attend patients, with separate teams for medical and cardiac patients evolving.

Each year, between one and three of UR's twenty-five pediatric and medicine-pediatric residents choose to specialize in pediatric critical care. Dr. Powers describes what it takes to be an effective intensivist: phenomenal attention to detail plus the ability to anticipate potential problems and respond quickly. "The most stressful aspect of critical care is multitasking and its potential for sensory overload. Things can change fast in the ICU. Our lifesavers are the remarkable nurses at the bedside who do so much to ensure good outcomes."

Career satisfaction for the intensivist comes not only from saving lives, but from being part of a close-knit group of physicians and nurses who, like soldiers in a MASH unit, are working toward a common goal. "We're like brothers and sisters," she says. "We always have each other's backs. When I suddenly learned that my husband had been seriously injured in a fall while out of state, a colleague immediately was on the phone booking my plane tickets and others were signing up to cover my schedule for the next week."

"Family comes first. That's our culture," says Dr. Powers. All the physicians in the division are parents; careful scheduling ensures they won't be "absent parents." When her son played high school basketball and football, Karen never missed a game. She also was president of the teams' booster club and served on the curriculum council for the town's schools. Help at home was essential, she notes. As part of a two-physician family, she's grateful for the financial luxury that made backup support possible, from either a nanny or an au pair.

Dr. Powers's pride in the growth of the division, her PICU colleagues, and the residents she has helped train is great. As is her gratitude for the support she has had from Dr. Elizabeth McAnarney, her longtime department chair. "Lissa has always had her pulse on our work and her support has been unending," she says. "To have a chairman appreciate your commitment and hard work means a lot."

Each year, about 1,200 PICU patients leave the hospital in better health than when they entered. For many, the critical care they received was life-saving, thanks to physician-intensivists like Dr. Karen Powers, who not only thrive in this high-energy, crisis-packed environment but inspire new generations of PICU physicians.

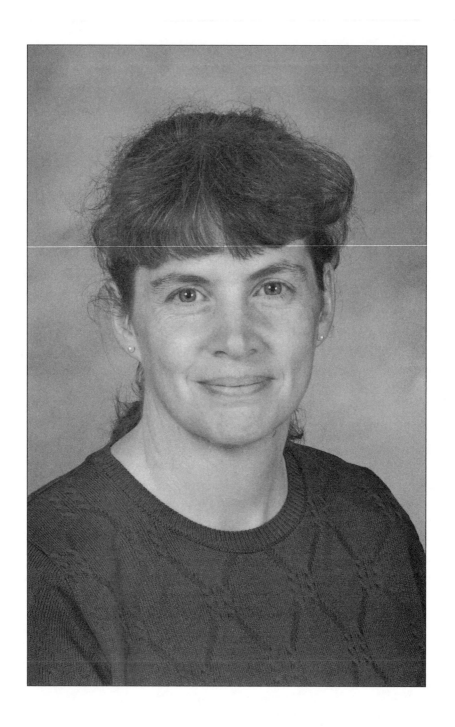

Chapter Twenty-Five

GLORIA S. PRYHUBER, MD

Gloria Pryhuber grew up in Hobart, a village of six hundred people amid the lush dairy farms of New York's Delaware County. Her family owned the local appliance store, and, as her father's fourth daughter, Gloria was his home-grown apprentice. "I loved going with him on service calls, watching as he installed washing machines or fixed clogged dishwashers, TVs on the fritz or refrigerators that warmed instead of cooled," she says. "I also was his chief equipment finder, maybe because I could understand what he wanted before he said it."

Young Gloria was so efficient, so energetic, the family began calling her "George," adapting a phrase then in common use—"Let George do it"—to describe a multitalented, indispensable helper.

Today, "Dr. Gloria" is a neonatologist and a pulmonary disease specialist who oversees two multimillion-dollar NIH research projects within UR Pediatrics. With colleagues at health centers across the country, she studies the data on infants (even those in utero) and young children with respiratory morbidity, looking for ways to improve outcomes.

Dr. Pryhuber also oversees the $6 million UR portion of the $20 million Molecular Atlas of Lung Development Program (LungMAP), an NIH-funded, multi-institutional undertaking. Because little is known about how human lung structures are molecularly programmed to develop, bioscientists are creating a library of tissue samples taken at various stages of lung growth. Two- and three-dimensional models developed from the samples, researchers hope, will help determine ways to fight common respiratory conditions, such as lung diseases of prematurity, asthma, pneumonia, cystic fibrosis, adult bronchitis, and emphysema.

In the Pryhuber Laboratory on the fourth floor of the University of Rochester Medical Center, technicians working in a protected environment prepare human bio specimens from blood, urine, and saliva for RNA and DNA testing, as well as tissue samples from umbilical cords and lungs donated by families from infants too frail to survive to be candidates for organ transplantation.

As a specialist in problems of premature infants, Dr. Pryhuber also teaches and mentors research fellows and PhD candidates and advises undergraduate students in career opportunities. In addition, each summer she sponsors and mentors students from Strong Children's Research Program, young people from the community who are interested in either medicine, medical technology, or both as a career.

"George," as you can see, is still doing it. Only now she's working within a national arena and on a powerfully human scale.

Life in Hobart was good, Gloria (then Gloria Salvini) says. With the Catskill Mountains and west branch of the Delaware River within easy reach, hiking adventures were balanced by visits with school friends who were part of Delaware County's thriving dairy farming culture and 4-H. The home family farms were hard work then but a great education. "I never learned that I couldn't do anything," she says. Though her high school was small—fifty students in her class—there were plenty of opportunities. Gloria played sports, was a cheerleader, and volunteered for the local ambulance corps. An admired older sister, now an ENT (ear, nose, and throat) surgeon in Texas, and good science teachers no doubt helped shape the young girl's future.

As for college, Gloria picked Cornell University in Ithaca. Her intention: to be a veterinarian and to attend Cornell's College of Agriculture and Life Sciences, one of the best in the nation. Once enrolled, Gloria discovered she could blend liberal arts *and* premed courses—and at a bargain price. "The Ag

School," as it was called then, was part of New York State's public university system, thus providing savings for medical school.

Was there a gender bias during the late 1970s? "Absolutely!" says Pryhuber. "There was a lot of talk about women being at Cornell to get their MRS Degrees. But I never allowed that kind of talk to stand in my way. I was 'George' and didn't know I couldn't do anything, so it just didn't matter!" While she acknowledges multiple mentors at Cornell, all served primarily as listening posts. "I needed mostly someone to listen as I charted my own path," she recalls. In a biology lab at Cornell, measuring testosterone effects in chickens, Gloria met Keith Pryhuber, the man who would soon become her husband. In 1981, she graduated from Cornell University with a Bachelor of Science degree, with distinction, and embarked with friends on a whirlwind tour of Europe. Back home again in Hobart, she finished the summer working at the local pill-packaging plant and lifeguarding at the community pool.

And then it was on to medical school and residency at Upstate Medical Center in Syracuse. "Pediatrics captured my imagination, not surprising maybe as the frequent babysitter and one who entertained the younger kids every holiday. My most meaningful mentor during my residency years," Gloria recalls, "was Dr. James A. Pollack, a pediatrician, a physician of children, with all his heart and soul. He taught me what it means to care for families and children, meeting them where they need you to be."

Her interests then turned to the youngest and smallest both to be able to help them but also because of fascination with the ever-changing physiology and technical aspects of neonatology. "A fellowship in neonatal-perinatal medicine at Cincinnati Children's Medical Center, with the opportunity to learn skills needed to pursue a laboratory research career, fostered by Dr. Jeffery Whitsett, was both life changing and the most logical direction for me."

After six years and with a fresh NIH grant in her pocket, Dr. Pryhuber came to Rochester where she says she found "a perfect combination of support and freedom." "Over the years, since arriving in 1994, I looked for collaborators, and found them, easily ... men and women, clinicians and investigators, MDs and PhDs. I think I've been able to blend my experiences in fixing machines and in medicine and science to enable myself and others to do more, understand better." Gloria also credits the support of her husband, Keith, a rheumatologist in private practice, and her two children, Jennifer and Andrew, for giving her a life outside of medicine and science. The frozen November camping trips with the Boy Scouts, sitting for hours (and hours) at wrestling tournaments for short minutes of pride, working on piano and voice lessons, getting to know other parents, and contributing to the community in small ways of leadership in Scouts and school are memories forever.

> I do still wonder about "life-work balance." But I don't think that's measured in time but in quality. Maybe better balance would have been more comforting to my family? Wish we'd done more dance . . . but they have always known that I do what has meaning to me because it is important to others and I think (hope) that has had good meaning in shaping their lives too. Jennifer studied at the NYU Tisch School of the Arts but then decided she wanted to "give back more" and is now an excellent registered nurse at the Mayo. Andrew is an adventurer, a whiz at math and a terrific, thoughtful, motivating teacher-type in graduate school. Where the children will go and what they will do remains something yet of a mystery but I know they will take satisfaction in doing it well. My husband? Well, he loves chopping wood; retirement in the Adirondacks will eventually, before too long, suit us both well.

Dr. Pryhuber maintains the same "can-do" attitude and dedication learned as a child in upstate New York in everything she undertakes. Her gentle nature, her deep intelligence and knowledge, and her kindness provide the perfect mentoring for the young.

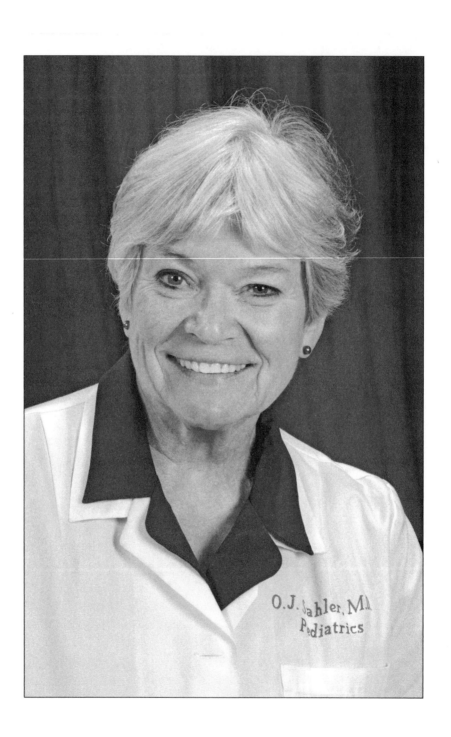

Chapter Twenty-Six

OLLE JANE (O. J.) Z. SAHLER, MD

The father of modern medicine, Sir William Osler, may have said it first: "One of the first duties of the physician is to educate." Dr. O. J. Sahler has created a national model of how to put Osler's dictum into action.

Dr. Sahler's work as founding president of the Council on Medical Student Education in Pediatrics (COMSEP) and the Alliance for Clinical Education (ACE) of the Association of American Medical Colleges (AAMC) has spread the work she began at the University of Rochester during the '70s and '80s throughout medical schools across the United States and Canada.

It may never have happened, however, if a brusque former chair of pediatrics hadn't ordered Sahler to take on two jobs for which, at the time, and as a new faculty hire, she felt unsuited. "I want you to direct the department's clerkship [its medical student education program]," he told her. "And I want you to get involved in computer-based education." That order seemed to lead off-course for a woman who had graduated from URMC with distinction and who had her eye fixed on a research career. (As for using computers, like most Americans at that time, she was a novice.) When Sahler voiced her concern, the chair said, "I've told you what I need you to do. Use the clerkship as your laboratory." She did.

That challenge—unwelcome, but inescapable—led to a career with important implications for pediatric medical education across the nation. It also led Dr. Sahler into the multiple worlds of psychiatry, oncology, pain management, integrative medical practice, and the dark topic of grieving families facing the death of a child.

"When I was a child, I knew what I was going to do when I grew up," Dr. Sahler says, with a smile. "I was going to be a nun, a missionary, and a teacher." Then at school one day, her eighth-grade homeroom teacher said: "Oh, not a doctor, like your father?" Sahler's father, a medical generalist in those days before the proliferation of subspecialties, was on the Yale University faculty. "A light bulb went off in my head that day," says Sahler. "I thought, 'Maybe I *could* do that.'"

Young Olle Jane was accepted at Radcliffe College, and like many of her fellow women students, she took most classes across the Cambridge Commons at Harvard, where she majored in biochemical sciences, graduating in 1966. Her parents, her father especially, were ambivalent about her plan to go to medical school; years earlier, a young woman in her father's medical school class at Yale, overwhelmed, had committed suicide; a second woman dropped out.

Sahler applied to only one medical school: the University of Rochester, a school rated highly by one of her father's physician-friends. O. J. believed she would need a medical degree if she were to undertake the human research that interested her. Assigned during her interview in Rochester to meet with the chair of the Department of Biochemistry, Dr. Elmer Stotz, she was awe-struck in his presence as she told him, "Dr. Stotz, I've read your papers!" Rochester, it seemed, was the right place for her.

Sahler was one of two women in her class of seventy-five students; six more would matriculate during the following three years. Yes, there were a few gender-unfriendly comments, such as "Oh, it's you who kept my [male] friend out of medical school. You'll just get married and never practice."

Never mind. Sahler worked hard, and found inspiration in her year-out program working with renowned behavioral pediatrician Dr. Stanford B. Friedman and two of the University of Rochester Medical Center's great humanists, Dr. John Romano and Dr. George Engel. In 1971, Dr. Sahler received her medical degree "with distinction in research."

That fall, when O. J. left Rochester to begin her pediatric residency training at Duke University, she was not traveling alone. With her was her new husband, Carl Sahler, a Princeton graduate who also had just received his UR medical degree, in addition to a PhD in cellular physiology at Roswell Park Cancer Institute at the University at Buffalo. Both, fortunately, "matched" at Duke University, O. J. in pediatrics and "Chip" in internal medicine. Newly integrated at that time, Duke's social environment as well as its approach to medical education was very different from what the Sahlers had experienced in Rochester—"less emphasis on the biopsychosocial aspects of care and a more hard-science based curriculum," O. J. recalls. Together, the two training styles made a complete whole.

In 1973, when the Sahlers had completed two years of residency, the country was still at war in Vietnam. At that time, all male doctors were required to be available for active military duty. O. J.'s voluntary enlistment meant her husband might have preferential treatment as to his posting.

Captain O. J. Sahler, USMC, spent the years from 1973 to 1975 as staff pediatrician at Silas B. Hays Army Hospital in Fort Ord, California. The experience would be transformational. As part of her work in a general pediatrics clinic, she began working with a child who had behavioral problems. "I wanted to do a school visit," she recalls, hoping to better understand the source of the trouble. "We've been waiting for someone like you," the hospital's child psychiatrist told her. This involvement with children at the biopsychosocial level would become a major focus of her career.

In 1975, the Sahlers, having fulfilled their military obligations, arrived back in Rochester. O. J.'s experience at Fort Ord led to a fellowship at the University of Rochester in behavioral/developmental pediatrics and child/adolescent psychiatry. Her seminal work in these areas would be supported by one of her career-long mentors, Dr. Elizabeth McAnarney, then chief of the Division of Adolescent Medicine and later chair of the Department of Pediatrics.

O. J. was also seven-months pregnant. Unable to scrub the far corners of the shower in their apartment because of her greatly expanded waistline, and married to a man whose cleaning prowess "didn't include bathrooms," O. J. hired help—a step she highly recommends to those entering a workforce that demands hard work and long hours.

Brian was born in 1975. He and his family now live in Portland, Oregon, where he teaches high school mathematics and AP (advanced placement) statistics. Catherine was born in 1978. She and her family live in Lima, New York, where she writes grants and conducts program evaluations for non-profit agencies.

It was about this time that the then-chair of pediatrics chose Sahler to direct the school's six-week pediatric clerkship; she would be the first woman at the medical school to be a clerkship director. The chair also laid down those previously mentioned mandates for her employment: In addition to leading the clerkship, she must develop a computer-based teaching program for the clerks and introduce it to an often-skeptical audience. "I had a 48-K Apple computer that I didn't understand," she says, smiling wryly in retrospect. Fortunately, help arrived at that moment in the form of a recently recruited faculty member in the medical education section of the dean's office who had a PhD in computer science. The computer course they developed was marketed nationally; it was so successful that the prototype was modified for use with nursing and dental students.

As Dr. Sahler watched each year's group of medical students work their way through their clerkship—interacting with physicians and nurses, seeing young patients, and meeting families deep in worry and grief—she became aware of a problem. Most children in hospitals were desperately ill; some would never get better. She realized that for some young medical students, still close to their own childhood, tragedy was too near and too constant. Could they bear the burden the profession demands? She decided to break the pattern of a solely hospital-based clerkship. After all, most children *do* get better. Why not include an outpatient component, where students could see the joy of taking care of children who had simpler, less threatening problems?

Making changes in a national institutionalized program like the pediatric clerkship is not easy. With support from another former chair of pediatrics, Dr. Robert Hoekelman, Sahler made that change happen, and Rochester's dual inpatient/outpatient–based clerkship became the first of its kind in the nation. She was gratified soon after to see the number of UR medical students who chose to specialize in pediatrics rise from four to eleven, in a medical school class of seventy-five.

Over the months during the 1980s, as radical change in the clerkship was underway, Sahler was consulting with heads of clerkships at medical schools across the country. "Rather than communicate one at a time, why shouldn't we be working together to create a set of national standards?" she wondered. The result: The Council on Medical Student Education in Pediatrics (COMSEP), now active across the US and Canada. Its founding president: Dr. O. J. Sahler. Her work—and her reputation—grew in 1993 when she also became the founding chair of the Alliance for Clinical Education (ACE).

Career changes that may seem rich with possibilities on occasion may come up short. In 1995, Dr. Sahler left Rochester for two years to become the director of the Department of Education at the national offices of the American Academy of Pediatrics in Chicago, where she led the effort to introduce the online version of the journal *Pediatrics*. At the same time, she became the principal investigator of an international multi-institutional research project funded by the National Cancer Institute to develop coping tools for mothers of children newly diagnosed with cancer. "After a time, I realized I had too many irons in the fire," she says; also, the back-and-forth to Rochester two weekends a month began to take its toll. Her decision to return home can stand as a lesson to young people: it's never a mistake to change course—when the cost of staying that course is too high.

Important new opportunities opened soon after Sahler returned to Rochester. She became part of a writing team for a Leadership Education in Adolescent Health (LEAH) grant, a project she served for fifteen years. Her interest in psychosocial oncology also continued to grow; she has led the department's Psychosocial Oncology Research and Education Program for more than twenty years and its Long-Term Childhood Cancer Survivors Program for more than twelve years.

Shortly after her return to Rochester, Sahler began a partnership with the Music Therapy Program at Nazareth College, one of whose purposes is to support non-pharmacologic management of painful procedures and anxiety. She now uses her training in biofeedback at the Adolescent Medicine Clinic to relieve young patients with chronic pain syndromes. As a member of the Pediatric Palliative Care team, she helps families and providers consider the wide range of options available for symptom management.

Dr. Sahler's editorial and authorial interests began as early as her fellowship years, when she convened a two-day conference in Rochester that focused solely on children and death, the first such conference worldwide. Subsequently she edited *The Child and Death* (1978), based on the papers given at the conference. In 1981, she and Dr. Elizabeth McAnarney co-authored *The Child from Three to Eighteen*; she also is the senior editor of *The Behavioral Sciences and Health Care*, now published in its fourth edition.

In 2012, Dr. Sahler became the principal investigator/project manager of a contract from NIH's Pain Consortium, the Rochester Area Collaborative Center of Excellence for Pain Education. This is one of only twelve centers across the nation, the focus of which is the responsible use of pharmacologic and non-pharmacologic approaches to pain management. Chaired by Dr. Sahler, the group links faculty from the URMC, St. John Fisher College in Pittsford, New York, and the New York Chiropractic College in Seneca Falls, New York.

Recently, the MAGIC (Media, Arts, Games, Interaction, and Creativity) Center at the Rochester Institute of Technology joined the center to develop innovative software to enhance learner engagement in online educational modules.

Dr. Sahler's passionate interest in education has led to leadership roles in her community, both on the Board of Education for the Canandaigua City School District for twenty-one years and as a member of the Wayne-Finger Lakes

Board of Cooperative Educational Services (BOCES) Board for more than twenty years. "Forty years of working with adolescents has shown me how children can be either adversely affected or empowered by their school experience," she says. She works to make the public aware of the growing value of BOCES's skills-based courses, a complementary educational model that can lead to satisfying, economically rewarding technical careers that carry high community value.

Dr. Sahler has some useful advice for young people embarking on a life in medicine. For those already in medical school who are looking to climb the academic ladder, her own career may be a helpful model. "Reaching out beyond the walls of your own institution is important," she says. "To make my longstanding NIH-sponsored pediatric oncology research more meaningful, I needed a sample size [a patient group] broader and larger than I could find in Rochester alone. So, I turned to the Children's Hospital of Los Angeles, the St. Jude Children's Research Hospital in Memphis, the University of Texas MD Anderson Cancer Center in Houston, as well as children's cancer centers in many other cities." More and more, medicine means partnering.

"Seize the opportunity—wherever you find it," Dr. Sahler advises. "The end product may not be clear at the time, but [if you follow the clues] things may well fall into place." For O. J. Sahler, each path she has entered has expanded, leading her into new territory. The result: a career rich in subject matter and rich in consequences—for her, her colleagues, her many trainees, and for thousands of patients.

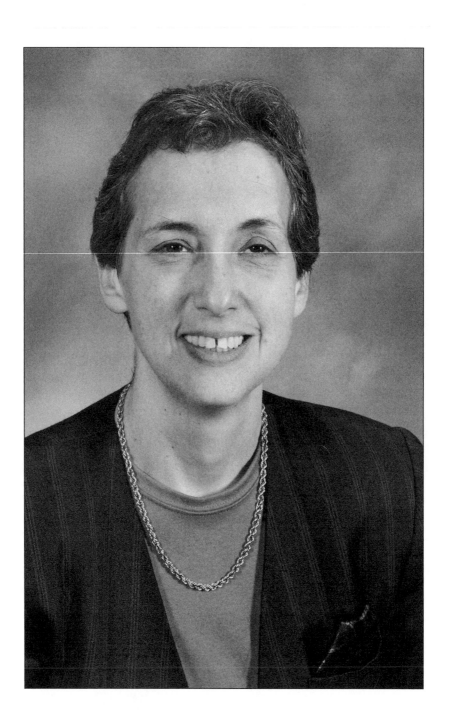

Chapter Twenty-Seven

Nina F. Schor, MD, PhD

Nina Schor's love of research began in the laboratory at Benjamin Cardozo High School on a quiet, tree-lined street in Bayside, Queens. There, at one of the nation's finest secondary schools, the talented young pianist discovered the wonder of scientific inquiry. "My experience in that lab gave me a sense of how exciting research could be," she says. "It was an intensely social, strongly interpersonal space, and very inspirational. I realized how much I enjoyed being in that lab, working with other kids who were drawn to science."

By 2017, nearly half a century later, Dr. Nina Schor was known nationally as a leader of one of the nation's premier pediatric programs. A career that began at Yale, Rockefeller, and Harvard took Schor upward through leadership roles at the University of Pittsburgh to the University of Rochester. There, during her tenure as the seventh chair of the Department of Pediatrics and Pediatrician-in-Chief, Dr. Schor raised the department to an historic new level, as measured by both size and funding.

Dr. Schor has had a major role in recent years, with chair emerita Dr. Elizabeth McAnarney, in developing Rochester's nearly $200 million Golisano Children's Hospital, a keystone of pediatric care for western New York, which opened in 2015. An important aspect of her leadership role in planning for the new hospital and its successful capital campaign was pointed out by University of Rochester Medical Center CEO Mark Taubman, MD: "(Nina) inspired trust in our families, physicians, and donors at a time when we very much needed community support."

One of the leading fundraisers in the history of the Department of Pediatrics, Dr. Schor helped UR Pediatrics's assets grow to $17 million in NIH funding; among its peers, it currently stands fifteenth in the nation in federal support. Add up all the department's research funds and contracts and funding for 2016 soared to $27.5 million. Dr. Schor herself has had continual federal funding throughout her career, support that has enabled her laboratory to do groundbreaking research on how to develop new strategies to treat tumors of the nervous system, including one of the most common childhood cancers, neuroblastomas.

Within the department, Dr. Schor has implemented a robust faculty development program, with faculty numbers growing from 110 to 170. The arrival of new faculty has made possible the founding of four new specialty divisions: Pediatric Sleep Medicine, Pediatric Allergy/Immunology, Pediatric Palliative Care, and Pediatric Hospital Medicine.

During her tenure as chair, Dr. Schor also oversaw the development of two important new centers. The Levine Autism Center brings together children with developmental disabilities and doctors with the expertise to help them and their families: developmental and behavioral pediatricians, child neurologists, and child psychiatrists. The Complex Care Center is designed to serve adults with disorders that began in childhood.

In 2017, Dr. Schor was awarded the John B. Hower Award, the highest honor given by the Child Neurology Society, the national organization for the subspecialty in which she is trained. The Hower Award joins the list of twenty-one other honors that she has received since her career began. She is a member of several professional organizations, including the American Academy of Neurology, the American Pediatric Society, the American Association for Cancer Research, and the American Association for the Advancement of Science, of which she was recently elected a Fellow.

As a committed research scientist who became a high-level administrator, Dr. Schor sees herself as a "big-picture person." She knows that most advances in medicine grow from seeds planted in medical laboratories here and around the world, and she's optimistic about the future. "Never before has the gap between biomedical research and clinical practice been so narrow," says Dr. Schor.

Under her guidance, the University of Rochester has enhanced its national reputation not only as a provider of top-quality care for children, but also as a training ground and supportive home for aspiring young scientists and clinicians. "I look at the academic physicians and physician scientists who come to Rochester with just a dream and fire in their belly and I see how they are bringing those dreams to fruition. That's what I'm most proud of," Dr. Nina Schor says of her eleven-year career in Rochester.

In 2018, Dr. Schor was appointed deputy director of the National Institute of Neurological Disorders and Stroke in Bethesda, MD.

Growing up in Queens, Nina Tabachnik was part of a family where business and the arts were richly blended. In those early days of room-size computers, her father, who had a doctoral degree in chemical engineering and physics, ran the national computer communications network for Mobil. Her mother, a buyer in Manhattan's garment center, was an actress and singer, both semi-professional avocations. Nina's sister had a successful career singing with opera companies in Santa Fe, New York, and Philadelphia. Nina herself is an accomplished pianist, and might have pursued a concert career—if not for that science class at Benjamin Cardozo high school.

At Yale University in the early 1970s, Nina found herself at home in the laboratories. "Yale was an incredible place," she says, "and through the breadth of its curricular elements, it allowed me to create my own course. I focused my research on biochemical questions. I learned tools there that I use even today as I study the three-dimensional structure of proteins, life's building blocks." She graduated *cum laude* in 1975 with a degree in molecular biophysics and biochemistry and with an honor perhaps unique to Yale: Scholar of the House, a program that allows the senior year to be spent entirely in independent study and research. "These were the Cold War years, yet our laboratories looked like a League of Nations, with postdocs from Mexico, Iran, and Turkey all working together cooperatively and becoming good friends," Dr. Schor recalls.

Nina spent the next six years studying at Rockefeller University, where she earned her doctoral degree in medical biochemistry (1980), and at Cornell University Medical School, where she received her medical degree (1981).

This was a heady time for the young graduate student. "If you met a snag in your research, everyone came together to help you solve the problem. It was instantly social."

Nina's internship and clinical residency years in pediatrics were spent in Boston at Boston Children's Hospital and Harvard Medical School. During her internship at Boston Children's Hospital, she says, she faced her steepest learning curve. "We had to learn by doing." At the bedsides of sick children, she worked to become comfortable making weighted decisions based on all available facts. Mentally marshaling information and carefully considering the pros and cons of each possible action, she sensed she was working at her highest level. "Even though I received my medical degree in 1981, it wasn't until a year later that I truly felt I was a doctor," she says. That sense of being secure in her knowledge was strengthened by the experience of teaching, sharing her new knowledge with medical students.

Boston would continue to be Dr. Schor's home for five years while she completed her residencies in pediatrics with Dr. M. E. Avery and in neurology with Dr. C. F. Barlow. "My intention in doing a child neurology residency instead of going straight into a postdoctoral or faculty research position was to ensure that my later research addressed the issues most critical to our understanding of neurological disease," she says.

It was in the laboratories at Harvard that Dr. Schor, the scientist, began the work that has inspired her research career: understanding the chain of events that results from sequential chemical changes in proteins—a sequence called "signal transduction"—and that underlies the development of tumors of the nervous system and neural diseases such as Alzheimer's and Parkinson's.

In 1986, Dr. Schor moved from Boston to Pittsburgh with her husband, neurophysiologist Robert Schor; the couple had married during Nina's second year of residency. Both had been offered faculty positions at the University of Pittsburgh, Nina as assistant professor of pediatrics and neurology.

Before leaving Harvard, Nina had questioned the wisdom of the move to Pittsburgh. The chair of pediatrics there thought it unwise for pediatricians to spend all of their time in research and not to do significant fractions of their time in the clinic. "Unless I had a lot of protected time, I couldn't collect the preliminary data I needed to get funding," she says. She was worried.

Luck, or fortune, would be with her. Michael Painter, MD, Pittsburgh's chief of child neurology and a key mentor in whose division she would work, viewed himself as her advocate in obtaining what she would need to be successful. "I explained my work on tumors in the nervous system and told him what I would need to continue," she says. "He believed in me—and he backed me up, going to the powers that be and speaking on my behalf." Her protected time was secured. By 2000, Dr. Schor held an endowed position in pediatric research within the University of Pittsburgh's Children's Hospital. Sometimes, she says, that's the best thing a mentor can do: believe in you.

Nina, of course, *did* often teach during those years in Pittsburgh (1986–2006). She was also reinventing herself, moving from the relatively small pond of the laboratory to the larger world that is Pittsburgh's medical center. Within that arena, she served as associate dean for medical student research and chief of the Division of Child Neurology, which at Pitt was housed within the Department of Pediatrics.

Three years after Nina and Robert arrived in Pittsburgh, they felt financially secure enough to begin a family and daughter Devra was born in 1989. Four years later, twin boys joined the family. (Devra is now a lawyer in California, providing legal services within the social sector. The twins, Jonathan and Stanford, are both MD/PhD students, one at Stanford University, the other at University of California, San Francisco. Former star athletes at Brighton High School, both also are talented musicians).

Music is also a lively part of Nina's world. In Pittsburgh, she played piano with a merry group of professional musicians whose klezmer band played gigs under the moniker, "The Hot Matzohs."

In September 2006, Dr. Nina Schor became the William H. Eilinger Chair of Pediatrics at the University of Rochester School of Medicine and Dentistry, Pediatrician-in-Chief at Strong Memorial Hospital (now Golisano Children's

Hospital), and professor of pediatrics and of neurology. A year later, she was named professor of neurobiology and anatomy and director of the PhD program in translational biomedical science.

With Dr. Schor's new position came invitations to talk about the current state of pediatrics at more than a dozen colleges and universities, including schools in Vermont, Cleveland, Maryland, Pittsburgh, Arkansas, California, Utah, and Boston. These honorific occasions, along with professional meetings with colleagues around the country, had a special importance: they were opportunities for her to help Rochester forge important connections with larger institutions.

Dr. Schor explains: Much medical research now takes place in highly focused "centers of excellence," including several at the University of Rochester. In order to achieve research depth and scale, research faculty need access to patient populations large enough to provide subjects who meet strict study specifications. Small or midsize departments, such as UR Pediatrics, can only achieve that depth and scale by partnering with larger institutions. Dr. Schor made strengthening those connections an important part of her mission.

Another critically important goal for the new chair was to increase funding to train aspiring doctors and to support the career development goals of the department's practicing physicians. During her many mentoring sessions with young faculty, Dr. Schor stressed the importance of taking time out from a busy schedule to set career goals and to find one or two faculty to talk with informally about both present work and future plans.

Of the dozens of early investigators who have been mentored by Dr. Schor, one might speak for all. "Nina has keen insights that reach beyond the boundaries of a single discipline," says Dr. Homaira Rahimi, assistant professor of pediatrics. "I'm a rheumatologist and Nina has a specialty in neurology, but she was able to show me where and how to make changes that are advancing my career. Her advice helped me obtain an important NIH award for early investigators. That's a big step forward."

In 2015, Dr. Schor was awarded the University of Rochester Medical Center's Faculty Academic Mentoring Award. That, and the recent Hower

Award honor from the Child Neurology Society are dear to Dr. Schor's heart. "The annual meetings of the Society are like family reunions," she says. "Ninety percent of those attending are doctors I've trained, doctors with whom I've trained, or doctors who trained me."

Research, leadership, family, community—all can be bound together within a single profession. Dr. Schor knows why her particular focus among that quartet—her work as a scientist—is important. "My research sits at the interface among and between fields, and it connects these fields in a unique way. Through this synergistic connection, all the components are energized so that the sum is greater than the parts. What I do best is juxtapose bodies of knowledge that influence one another. For example, the principles I use to design new treatments for neuroblastoma come not from neuroscience, not from cancer biology, but from basic science. It's important to remember that the principles we discover in basic science can—and will—inform our understanding of human neurodevelopment."

As Dr. Nina Schor looks back over her eleven-year tenure, she talks about the pleasures and stresses of leadership. She mentions again the feeling of community that enriches national meetings with her colleagues in child neurology. She found similar support and friendship during her years as department chair. "The collegiality among Rochester faculty stands at a level I've not found anywhere else," she says. "I've found that if the person who assumes leadership is comfortable with at least one or two of the disciplines held by her faculty, they will say, 'Welcome! You are one of us. We're all in this together.'"

For young people coming into pediatrics, Dr. Schor offers the advice that she has followed:

- Recognize what you love to do—and what you don't. Then surround yourself with people who excel at doing what you *don't* like to do.
- Identify your own strong suits and those of your team members. Design a working plan that plays to individual strengths and provides outside support for the analogous weaknesses.
- Listen well and read between the lines.
- Value all components and contributions.

- Listen and learn from everyone and everything.
- Thought without action is useless. Action without thought is worse.
- Development is forever.
- If you can't laugh at the person who looks back at you from the mirror, the ballgame is over.

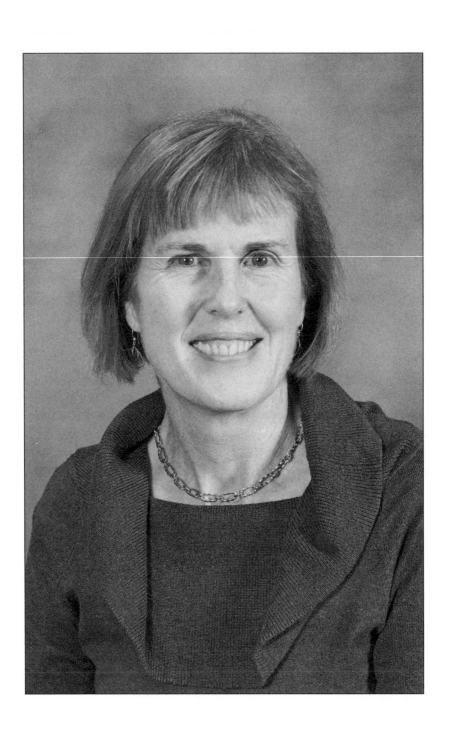

Chapter Twenty-Eight

MOIRA A. SZILAGYI, MD, PHD

It is easier to build strong children than to fix broken men.

—Frederick Douglass

Those words by Rochester's iconic abolitionist are written on the cover page of Dr. Moira A. Szilagyi's curriculum vitae. The message sounds a powerful chord that resonates throughout her career. As a national advocate for vulnerable children, Dr. Szilagyi broadcasts a warning that children in foster care are the "canary in the coal mine" for thousands of other children suffering from social-induced trauma. And she has spent years working to fix the problem.

"As a young pediatric clinician working within the county healthcare system, I realized we were seeing only the tip of the iceberg. A much larger population of children and adolescents never come to the attention of child welfare professionals," she says. "This is a micro-culture fraught with separation, loss, and uncertainty. Those youngsters who slip through the social network are often left alone to face multiple adversities." Her career goal became clear: she would find ways to help powerless children caught in a system not of their making.

As a new primary care pediatrician at the University of Rochester during the early 1990s, Moira went into action. She saw that children in foster care *and* their foster parents need support from professionals who understand the intricacies of the system. With a small staff and a shoestring budget, she turned a fledgling county clinic, Starlight Pediatrics, into a national model for pediatric services for children and adolescents in foster care. Monroe County children within that revolving world found at Starlight Pediatrics a secure and stable place, a medical home where they could talk with doctors and social workers trained to address their often complex problems. Perhaps just as important, Dr. Szilagyi found the money to build the program.

As Starlight's medical director, Moira brought together healthcare professionals from several disciplines to test and then implement the most effective ways to promote the health and resiliency of youngsters in foster care. She describes the challenge: "Aside from the strain of instability itself, anxiety and stress can have an adverse impact on children's physical health. So, while minding all this, our specialists must support foster parents in nurturing each child's unique personality and temperament. We need to help these children navigate transitions through new schools, new childcare settings, and the court process as comfortably as possible."

Dr. Szilagyi's career-long advocacy for children has had an impact at the highest national levels. In 2008, she worked with the American Academy of Pediatrics and thirty-seven other organizations to provide the policy foundation for the US Congress's passage of the most significant child welfare legislation in over a decade, the *Fostering Connections to Success and Increasing Adoptions Act*. Her book, *Fostering Health*, is the leading healthcare book on foster care; she led the development of the *Healthy Foster Care America* website, a widely used educational resource for healthcare and social welfare professionals and families. In addition to writing several AAP policy statements and technical reports that set the health agenda for children in foster care, she has collaborated with the federal government's Children's Bureau around health and mental health issues in the child welfare population.

In 2007, the AAP recognized Dr. Szilagyi's work with a major award recognizing her as "a pediatrician who has demonstrated clinical excellence, community action, and advocacy for children with unique care needs."

Moira's family moved to this country from Australia in the early 1960s, and her father found work as a bricklayer at a Ford Motor Company plant near Albany. At that time, the Ford Foundation offered two scholarships at each plant to children of employees: full tuition and three-quarters of the cost of the year's room and board. Competition was intense, but Moira was a winner. (Moira's father offered to buy her a car if, after working hard, she won.) "It was a miracle," says Moira. "No one in my family had ever gone to college."

She chose Siena College, a Catholic college in Loudonville, New York, whose programs in business and science were well-respected. "My parents were strict Irish Catholics," she says, "and in the wild sixties, Siena seemed like a safe harbor for an unsophisticated young woman like me. Siena's reputation for being theologically liberal wasn't a problem. My father always encouraged us to challenge our belief system," she says. Moira graduated from Siena as a chemistry major, valedictorian, and *summa cum laude.*

Moira arrived at the University of Rochester and began her postgraduate education in biochemistry, supported by a National Research Service Award and an Elon Huntington Hooker Fellowship. Moira was fortunate, she says, to be mentored by scientist Dr. Guido Marinetti, whose fellows were involved in lipid metabolism research. "Guido took me under his wing and he was very nurturing," she says. When she considered dropping out of the PhD program, his counsel helped change her mind. "All my friends then were medical students and their work sounded much more interesting than what I was doing," she says. "You don't want to lose your fellowship," Dr. Marinetti cautioned. "Remember, nothing you learn is ever wasted. Get your doctoral degree and *then* apply to medical school." Moira was awarded her doctoral degree in 1980.

Medicine as a career had never been a consideration for Moira. As a girl, she had little exposure to doctors. "I expected to be an elementary school teacher," she says. At Rochester, she had her first real exposure to the discipline of medicine—and found it fit her value system. She also met Peter Szilagyi, already a medical student. ("I knew I'd found a winner," she says.) The couple married between her first and second years. Unexpectedly, she says, she soon was pregnant, and nine months later Moira became the first woman at UR to have a child, a daughter, during medical school. She received her medical degree in 1984, and began her internship, working on a reduced schedule. The couple's second child, a son, was born during her internship. With support from the then-chair of pediatrics Dr. Robert Hoekelman, she was able to share her residency with a female classmate. ("We were probably the first such 'matched couple' in the country," she says.)

Although Moira searched for the right medical specialty that fit, Peter had long known that pediatrics was his calling. Things changed for Moira when she began her medical school rotation in pediatrics at the Rochester General Hospital Neonatal Intensive Care nursery. "I knew in the first hour that pediatrics is where I wanted to be, that this is where I belonged," she says.

Academic pediatricians strive to be skilled clinicians, researchers, and inspiring teachers. Moira honed these talents early in her career, first teaching chemistry at Nazareth College in Pittsford, New York. Later, as a clinical instructor in pediatrics at the University of Rochester Medical Center, she worked part-time in a Rochester primary care practice and at the juvenile offenders' detention center run by Monroe County Department of Health. In 1992, Dr. Szilagyi founded and became co-director of REACH, the regional medical referral center that evaluated suspected child abuse and neglect, a program initiated by the URMC Department of Pediatrics.

Dr. Szilagyi's connection with the county health department strengthened when, in 1990, she was appointed director of Starlight Pediatrics. "When Starlight began, little was known about the healthcare needs of children in foster care and what leads to success, or failure, for these children who face multiple adversities." At Starlight, over time, comprehensive pediatric, mental health, developmental, and dental care was integrated within this new medical home model. In 2009, Szilagyi obtained a $3.1 million New York State grant to construct a centralized medical home for children in foster care that became a national model. A second grant, this one for $1.3 million from the Centers for Disease Control, supported integration of the evidence-based practices that provided comprehensive care for Starlight children and adolescents.

Dr. Szilagyi's team of experts came from the Department of Pediatrics, Strong Behavioral Health, Mt. Hope Family Center (all representing the University of Rochester) and physicians and staff from Monroe County's Department of Human Services and Public Health. These collaborations provided a rich source of research data for team members. Dr. Szilagyi's own investigations were focused in three major areas:

- Developing interventions to systematically screen and manage developmental and mental health problems for children and adolescents in foster care.
- Implementing and evaluating healthcare standards for children in foster care.
- Translating evidence-based, promising interventions into real-world care of children in foster care, with attention to parenting education and developmental and mental healthcare.

Dr. Szilagyi stresses the importance of collaboration. "Early on, I learned that nothing good has come except through collaboration. I teach residents and others that advocacy for children involves a lot of 'P' words: Passion, Partnerships (often with others outside medicine), Persistence, Patience, and Politeness." For those in leadership positions, she stresses the importance of identifying and focusing on "Policy Points," steps needed to move the project forward. This kind of mentoring has been of help to dozens of mentees and has helped guide countless meetings both in and beyond academia.

Sandra Jee, MD, MPH, was a pediatric health services research fellow at the University of Michigan when she invited Dr. Szilagyi to serve as a visiting professor. Now an associate professor of pediatrics at the University of Rochester, Dr. Jee has co-written with her mentor many papers and book chapters on underserved children with behavioral health issues. "Moira is a thoughtful, insightful leader who knows how to support those of us who care for medically and socially complex patients," says Dr. Jee. "Just as important, she and her husband Peter have been role models for how to balance career and family. Moira has demonstrated to me, and many women, that it is possible to have a successful and fulfilling career while not always following a full-time work schedule. We have seen her carefully balance family and aspects of life that are beyond the prototypical academic aspirations. I am extremely grateful for her authenticity and willingness to be an atypical academic who has forged a unique path unlike most other women in academic medicine."

In 2014, Moira and Peter left Rochester for the University of California, Los Angeles, where she is now a professor of pediatrics and Peter is executive vice chair of the department. In collaboration with UCLA's Center for Healthier Children, Families & Communities and as a clinician caring for children at a Los Angeles County Hub Clinic, Moira continues to focus on identifying families and children at risk for poor outcomes and intervening early to build resistance to the deleterious effects of childhood adversity and trauma.

At UCLA, Moira participated in a Packard Foundation-funded grant to study the best ways to care for children with complex medical conditions. She currently spends two days a week in clinical work with children in foster care at Olive View-UCLA Medical Center and is involved in transforming this evaluation site into an integrated medical home model. In addition to her advocacy work at the national level, she leads a project that funds training for pediatricians across the country about the prevention and amelioration of the effects of psychological and other trauma on children.

Through the years, Dr. Szilagyi has been a frequent visiting professor and keynote speaker. Her honors and awards began in college when she was a Ford Foundation Scholar. Key among the long list is the Calvin C. J. Sia Community Pediatrics Medical Home Leadership and Advocacy Award from the AAP; the Dr. David Satcher Community Health Improvement Award; the W. Burt Richardson Lifetime Achievement Award from the Federation of Social Workers; and the 2016 Public Policy and Advocacy Award from the Academic Pediatric Association.

"My experience in Rochester has shaped both my life and my career," she says. "As young trainees, we could walk into any attending's office with a question and they would pay attention to us. We grew up steeped in the integrated medicine model that was unique to Rochester at that time. When we went out into the world it was eye-opening to realize that the skill sets we had learned were three and four decades ahead of the national curve."

Mentoring pediatric residents, fellows, and young faculty has been an important focus for Moira, both in Rochester and at UCLA.

Dr. Szilagyi has this advice for young women entering academic medicine:

- Follow your passion. It is much easier to go to work every day if you love what you are doing.
- If people tell you you're on the wrong track (as I was told on occasion), don't be discouraged. Do what you love.
- Don't let academic advancement be your chief goal. If you become good at what you love to do, advancement will follow.
- Pick a good partner. My husband has been my biggest support.

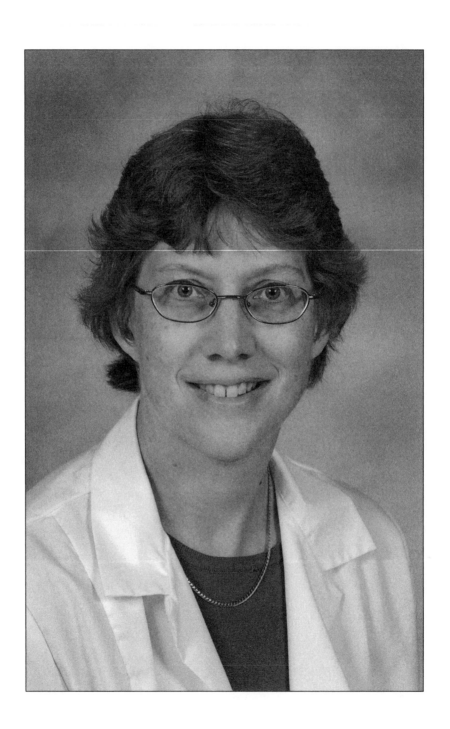

Chapter Twenty-Nine

KAREN Z. VOTER, MD

Dr. Karen Voter knows all of the medical complications that can steal children's breath, frighten them, complicate their lives, and even, tragically, shorten their lifespan. During a career that spans more than three decades, this pediatric pulmonary specialist has evaluated, diagnosed, and created treatment plans for hundreds of children with breathing disorders—from the infant born with a lung infection and a teenager with cystic fibrosis to a parent learning to provide home care for a child on a ventilator.

She is a member of a very select group of physicians. Across the nation there are only approximately one thousand board-trained pediatric pulmonary specialists available to treat hundreds of thousands of children who each year confront breathing issues. The challenges for these doctors are multiple. Not only are their young patients susceptible to all the lung diseases common to adults, but children's still-developing bodies and immune systems are especially vulnerable. Chronic cough, sleep apnea, asthma, lung infections, cystic fibrosis, lung diseases in premature infants: all are threats that Dr. Voter is prepared to meet after six years of specialty training and decades of clinical experience.

"The good news is that through research we've made great progress in treating pulmonary disease," Dr. Voter says. "Every year we have an answer to an old problem. New medications are available now that can clear clogged airways. Sometimes we even correct the basic defect. It's a very exciting time to be involved in the field."

"I always wanted to be a doctor," says Karen. She was immersed in the world of medicine during her childhood and adolescence when her father was chief of surgery at Johns Hopkins Hospital. She spent many Saturdays at the hospital with him and even had one summer job drawing blood from Hopkins patients. During those years she absorbed much of the clinical and teaching environment of a hospital and a sense of the dedication the profession of medicine demands. Her father went on to become vice provost for Health Affairs at the University of Michigan, which helped Karen become more aware of the importance of administrative achievements.

At Duke University, Karen majored in zoology and benefited, she says, from her small-size classes in cell biology and from hours spent in an equally small research laboratory. That research led to an opportunity: collecting specimens at the university's marine laboratory in Beaufort, North Carolina, where the young researcher studied the protein content of microtubules in sea urchins. Karen graduated *cum laude* from Duke in 1977.

At the University of Virginia School of Medicine in the late 1970s, one-third of Karen's classmates were women. Asked if she was aware of a gender-bias, she responds: "If there was [such a bias], I chose not to pay attention to it." The question of her medical specialization was open until she did a rotation in endocrinology at the University of North Carolina (UNC). She so enjoyed working with the children that it became clear that pediatrics would be her chosen field.

A joyous major life event occurred after graduation when Karen married William, the physics research associate she had fallen in love with at Duke. In the brief period between medical school and residency, the young couple was able to cross the country (by train) and honeymoon in California's wine country before Bill returned to Duke.

Dr. Voter says one of the most difficult periods in her life was transitioning between the first and second years of her residency; the second stressful time was becoming an attending physician after three years of fellowship. As for narrowing her focus within pediatrics, she gave much thought to general pediatrics, then decided that she would do better with a tighter focus. That focus would become pulmonary pediatrics.

Karen's three-year pediatric residency at UNC expanded into three years of pediatric pulmonary fellowship training. Her clinical research involved boys who had been treated for viral infections when they were young children. As teenagers, they were given pulmonary function tests, challenges that tested the lungs' response to increasing doses of inhaled nebulized methacholine, often used to determine the presence or absence of asthma. A second study involved measuring how fast particles moved in the airways of baby ferrets born without cilia in the lining of the trachea.

Her fellowship experience was strengthened by the support she received from two faculty mentors, Drs. Marianna Henry and Margaret Leigh. "Both were important in supporting my education, as well as enhancing my research and clinical skills," she says.

Pediatric pulmonology as a specialty was relatively new when Dr. Voter arrived at the University of Rochester in 1987 as an assistant professor, but pediatricians Dr. John Brooks and Dr. John McBride were building UR's reputation in what would soon become a burgeoning field. Their newly arrived colleague brought with her an important new skill: Dr. Voter had learned to do bronchoscopies at UNC while working with Dr. Robert Wood, professor of pediatrics and a leader in the test's development. Karen quickly was given two big responsibilities, as director of Strong Memorial Hospital's Pediatric Pulmonary Bronchoscopy Service and director of the Pediatric Pulmonary Function Laboratory, titles she still holds.

Her responsibilities continued to grow, as did the numbers of young patients coming into the hospital either as referrals from community pediatricians or as emergency patients. In 2002, Dr. Voter was appointed director of the Rochester chapter of the state's Cystic Fibrosis Newborn Screening Program. In 2015, she added another title: director of the Cystic Fibrosis Care, Teaching, and Research Center. She continues to direct both the screening program and the work of the Cystic Fibrosis Center. In 2017, she was appointed clinical director of the Division of Pediatric Pulmonology.

Currently, a monthly pie chart of Dr. Voter's working days would be divided this way: 70 percent patient care, 20 percent teaching, and 10 percent research. Her clinical responsibilities include evaluating all new patients and those with complex conditions who depend upon ventilators and live at home. Her students include those in medical school, residents, nurses, dental students, and pulmonary fellows. Once a year she teaches students in the Physician's Assistant Program at Rochester Institute of Technology (RIT).

Working with Dr. Voter to provide patient care are three nurse practitioners as well as colleagues from related specialties. "I'm proud of the fact that I've built collaborative relationships with cardiologists, neonatologists, and those who treat ear, nose, throat, sleep disorders, and other aerodigestive conditions." The pulmonary hypertension team is evidence of one of these important collaborations.

"Dr. Voter early on helped build the Department of Pediatrics's pulmonology program," says Distinguished University Professor and former chair of pediatrics Dr. Elizabeth McAnarney. "She is one of our most skilled and devoted clinicians and teachers. She is indefatigable in her professional devotion to her patients, their families, and to her colleagues." A member of the American Thoracic Society and the American Academy of Pediatrics, Dr. Voter's name is listed in "Best Doctors in America" and the "Consumers Research Council Guide."

Karen Voter has succeeded in combining work and family, and she gives much of the credit to her husband and to the cherished daycare provider who now, years later, continues to join the family for all major holidays. The Voters' three sons are Allen, an RIT graduate who owns a small computer consulting business in Kentucky; Andrew, who is working on his MD and PhD degrees at the University of Wisconsin; and Brian, a junior at Cornell University.

In a reflective moment, Karen talks about the challenges of combining work as a busy physician with family life. "What has worked for me is focusing on my most important goals which, over time, have narrowed into seeking peace and joy," she says. "What doesn't work is comparing myself to other people.

Too often that leads to guilt and fear." Throughout her life, Karen says she has been supported by her religious faith, a dedication that leads her to see the best in other people.

For children who struggle with breathing problems, the importance of work being done in clinic, classroom, and laboratory by Dr. Voter and her colleagues, here and around the world, deserves both support and high praise.